First Aid Manual for Chemical Accidents

The recommendations for emergency treatment found in this volume are based on procedures developed by recognized authorities and from the extensive experience of a major chemical producer. Nevertheless, the users of this first aid manual must realize that first aid techniques are constantly being improved and that the general standards for the health and safety of individuals are being raised. It is necessary that the book's users be trained to distinguish correctly the different symptoms of intoxication described in this book, that they be fully qualified to render first aid treatment, and that they remain current with the latest developments in first aid treatment. This manual is not to be construed as a substitute for any legal practice. In any case, the author, editor, publisher, or the publisher's agents shall not be liable or responsible in any manner whatsoever for any errors or omissions in this book, or for the use of the contents of this book.

First Aid Manual for Chemical Accidents

for Use with Nonpharmaceutical Chemicals

Compiled by

Marc J. Lefèvre, M.D.

Hygienist, Toxicologist, Medical Adviser,
Head of the Central Toxicological Service
of the Central Personnel Department of
SOLVAY & Cie, S.A., Brussels

English-language edition
edited by

Ernest I. Becker, Ph.D.

Professor of Chemistry, University of
Massachusetts, at Boston; American
Chemical Society's Committee on Chemical
Safety (former chairman) and Division
of Chemical Health and Safety
(former secretary-treasurer)

Dowden, Hutchinson & Ross, Inc.
Stroudsburg Pennsylvania

Translated from the French original by LAPORTE INDUSTRIES, LTD

Library of Congress Catalog Card Number: 80–17518
ISBN: 0–87933–336–7

82 3 4 5
Manufactured in the United States of America.

Library of Congress Cataloging in Publication Data

Lefèvre, Marc J
First aid manual for chemical accidents.
Translation of Manuel de premiers soins d'urgence.
1. First aid in illness and injury. 2. Industrial accidents. 3. Industrial toxicology. I. Becker, Ernest I., 1918– II. Title [DNLM: 1. Accidents, Occupational—Prevention and control—Handbooks. 2. First aid—Handbooks. 3. Toxicology—Handbooks.
WA465 M294]
RC963.3.L4313 615.9'08 80–17518
ISBN 0–87933–336–7

Distributed world wide by Academic Press,
a subsidiary of Harcourt Brace Jovanovich,
Publishers.

CONTENTS

CONTENTS

Editor's Preface

Of the many first aid manuals on the market, none is dedicated totally to first aid at the workplace in which industrial chemicals are used. First aid for chemical accidents requires specific, quick, correct action to obviate or minimize potentially serious, harmful effects. An easily readable, handily indexed source book has been necessary. It is to this need that the *First Aid Manual for Chemical Accidents* directs itself.

Conceived and extensively tested in Solvay & Cie, S. A., it was expanded in scope beyond that required by a single company and carried to its present state by Dr. Marc J. Lefèvre. Included among those for whom it is intended are: supervisors of manufacturing operations in which chemicals are used, first aiders, workers in manufacturing, firemen, chemists, laboratory supervisors, chemical engineers, and farm workers. Thus, it will find use as a pocket guide and quick reference in factories, laboratories, on farms, in forests, and wherever industrial solvents, insecticides, commercial chemicals, fertilizers, and chemical intermediates are found.

The text provides a source of clear information on the proper treatment of persons exposed to toxic levels of industrial chemicals. Following five pages describing the manual and its use, there is the GOLDEN RULE, followed by 16 pages of an index of almost 500 industrial products and their most common synonyms. For each compound, section references to toxicology (white pages), first aid procedures in cases of inhalation (yellow pages), ingestion (green pages), skin contact (pink pages), and eye contact (blue pages) are given. This easily perceived indexing scheme makes the information quickly available; but, of course, the manual should be read as part of one's training prior to working in dangerous atmospheres.

It is hoped that this manual will make the work of the first aider more effective and thus minimize or obviate the trauma normally associated with industrial chemical accidents.

In the United States, the National Institute of Occupational Safety and Health (NIOSH) recommends standards for exposure to compounds in the workplace to the Occupational Safety and Health Administration (OSHA), which then promulgates and enforces them. A list of relevant publications appears in Appendix B.

Since time is of the essence in emergencies, masculine pronouns are used throughout this manual for succinctness and are intended to refer to both females and males.

ERNEST I. BECKER

Compiler's Preface

This manual of first aid is not the work of only one physician, but of a whole staff.

Without the bibliographical references, books, and data that SOLVAY & C° has provided to its Department of Toxicology, this manual would have been left as a draft or a project in a drawer.

The first French edition is out of print.

I express all my gratitude for the really valuable assistance to all the people of SOLVAY & Cie, S.A., Brussels, of LAPORTE INDUSTRIES, LTD and of THE SOLVAY AMERICAN CORPORATION who collaborated on the issue of this first, newly revised English-language edition. The English translation and medical terminology have been reviewed by me.

M. J. LEFÈVRE, M.D.

Compiler's Preface

Introduction

I. THE IMPORTANCE OF THE FIRST AIDER'S ROLE

Books and pamphlets on emergency treatment are too often intended exclusively for toxicologists, doctors, or medical officers who have years of experience and a thorough knowledge of biochemistry, clinical pathology, toxicology, and diagnosis. Authors also assume that these practitioners have adequate medical equipment and drugs available.

Nothing has been written specifically for the first aider, the foreman, or the laboratory assistant. We wished to fill this gap. We therefore took as our model "Gassing Casualties," written by Dr. Amor of ICI during the bombing of London in 1940, and published in 1952 and 1957 by the Association of British Chemical Manufacturers.

This *First Aid Manual for Chemical Accidents* was conceived, planned, and written for persons other than doctors: foremen, first aiders, production workers, firemen, chemists, heads of laboratories, chemical engineers, and agricultural workers.

These are the people—in the factory, on the production line, in the laboratory, on farms or in forests—who could suddenly be called on to render assistance to a fellow worker or a stranger—the victim of poisoning, mistake, or accident.

They will have to move the victim to a safe place and revive or help him until the arrival of a physician or nurse, who have the authority and experience to provide adequate medical treatment. The first aider must, however, have administered appropriate first aid without delay so that the victim is alive when the physician or nurse arrives.

It is, in fact, the first aider's duty and responsibility to give the

Since time is of the essence in emergencies, masculine pronouns are used throughout this manual for succinctness and are intended to refer to both females and males.

alarm, to protect himself suitably (appropriate mask, apron, gloves, goggles), to remove the victim from danger and the contaminated area, to notify the medical services,* to take charge of the victim, and to calm and comfort him, with a view to minimizing the consequences of the accident.

II. DESCRIPTION OF THE MANUAL

A. Introduction

This is the text you are now reading.

B. Vital Equipment

Equipment should be selected according to the types of hazards that are most likely to be encountered in plants or elsewhere. Apart from the standard means of protection (appropriate masks, aprons, gloves, goggles, etc.) and according to the nature of the hazardous products being handled, this equipment should include a spoon; one or two drinking glasses; a kidney basin; a bucket; two blankets, preferably of wool; a stretcher, cot, or bed; a sink with hot and cold water faucets; a cold or, preferably, luke-warm shower; soap; towels; a pair of strong scissors; a simple BROOK airway or an AMBU-type apparatus. For serious cases, an oxygen cylinder with control valve and mask should be included or, better still, a safety resuscitating apparatus similar to the PULMOTOR, PNEOPHORE, PORTON, or AIROX.

Apart from a few standard pharmaceutical products (70% alcohol, ether, cotton wool, dry dressing, lime water, calcined magnesia, mineral oil or Nujol, sodium sulfate, etc.), first aid never requires medicinal preparations. Foodstuffs such as milk or fresh eggs are often recommended. Powdered milk or eggs can be kept very well for a long time in hermetically sealed cans.

*See inside front cover of your telephone directory for the nearest Poison Information Center or Poison Control Center.

C. Index

This alphabetical list gives the common names and some synonyms of almost 500 substances most often encountered in the chemical industry and in agriculture.

In order to avoid making the index unmanageable, we have not included a full list of all synonyms and have deliberately refrained from dealing with pharmaceutical substances proper.

The numbers following the chemical names in the index refer the first aider to the symptoms (**white** pages) and advise first aid according to the types of contact with the substances (**yellow**, **green**, **pink**, and **blue** pages).

D. Table of Symptoms (white pages)

In these **white** pages we have grouped together in "families" substances that have more or less similar action, assigning a section number to each family.

1. At the top of the page—names of the products covered
2. Next—concise information regarding any physical or toxic properties
3. Finally—a list of symptoms in the most usual or probable order in which they appear for the various types of contact, with references to the colored pages for first aid.

These lists include the more serious SYMPTOMS **that would be observed if the victim were given no first aid and no subsequent medical treatment**. This is why most of the descriptions of serious poisoning terminate with the words "coma" and "death."

At this point, one must make a comparison: If a child falls into water or an adult is caught in quicksand, death will inevitably put an end to their vain efforts, their anguish, and their cries for help if no outside aid reaches them. A hand, a cloth, or a branch held out can quickly save their lives or prevent any serious consequences; the accident becomes an incident and eventually an anecdote. But then it is necessary that the person seeing the tragedy, the first aider in this case, acts quickly and coolly. Reading the descriptions should not, therefore, provoke panic, but instead the determination to act quickly and calmly in order to prevent the most tragic result.

E. First-Aid Instructions (yellow, green, pink, and blue pages)

The colored pages list the first aid to be given in the prescribed order, before the arrival of the physician, depending on the patient's condition and the effects of the poison.

— the **yellow** pages refer to poisoning by INHALATION

— the **green** pages, to poisoning via the digestive tract by INGESTION or SWALLOWING

— the **pink** pages, to SKIN CONTACT

— the **blue** pages, to EYE CONTACT

Each of the colored pages repeats the list of substances for which the first aid given is valid.

In order to avoid any mistake, it is always important to verify whether the relevant chemical substance is listed at the top of the first-aid page consulted.

F. Appendix A

GENERAL INSTRUCTIONS IN CASE OF POISONING BY UNKNOWN CHEMICAL PRODUCTS.

The information in these pages is intended for cases where the exact chemical nature of the injuring substance is doubtful or unknown, for example, a person found unconscious or with evidence of splashing by a mixture of irritating substances.

G. Appendix B

U.S. GOVERNMENT PUBLICATIONS

Information concerning U.S. government publications relevant to some of the chemicals covered in this manual are listed.

H. Appendix C

GLOSSARY OF COMMERCIAL NAMES

Chemical names for commercial products listed in the index are given. The commercial names in the index are followed by an asterisk (*).

III. USE OF THE MANUAL

To be successful, first aid must be given without delay.

In cases where the substance that has caused the symptoms is not precisely known, one must judge

— from the external or organoleptic characteristics (that is, smell, appearance, viscosity, color, etc.) of the handled substances in order to determine the relevant substance;

— or from the state of the victim.

In such cases, consult **APPENDIX A** on page 211.

Generally, however, the substance responsible will be known. In this event

1. Look up the name of the substance in the index; this name is followed by several numbers that refer to the sections to be consulted;
2. First refer to the section number of the white pages given in the first column. Verify whether the symptoms roughly correspond to those described. If they do not, follow the general instructions given in **APPENDIX A** on page 211.
3. If they do, which is generally the case, look up the section number of the colored pages corresponding to the type of contact of the substance;
4. Quickly read the first aid to be administered on the appropriate colored page;
5. Abide by the advice given, follow the order laid down, and always remember to take the necessary precautions to protect yourself.

Do not forget that sometimes two poisonous effects may occur simultaneously or consecutively. For example,

a. Splashing with caustic soda lye may affect both the eyes and arms.

In this case, *the eyes must take first priority as far as speed of treatment is concerned.* Treat them first and then undress the victim under the shower. See the GOLDEN RULE, page 9.

b. A splash of chlorinated solvent soaks a trouser leg. A risk of inhalation can be secondarily associated with the skin contact. The first aider will take the appropriate action; he will remove the contaminated clothing to the open air and warn those around of the danger.

IV. CONCLUSIONS

The *First Aid Manual for Chemical Accidents* is written in clear, concise language; it is sometimes brief but only in order to save time. The aim is that it should be on hand always and everywhere to be consulted immediately. It is intended to contribute to saving lives, if possible, and, at least, to lessening the sufferings of victims of chemical accidents and minimizing aftereffects.

First aiders will, in this way, earn the gratitude of the people they have helped, the esteem of the medical profession, and, above all, they will cherish the unforgettable feeling of having unselfishly and properly helped a fellow man. We hope that this small work will be widely read and its message clearly understood.

GOLDEN RULE

Always treat
the most urgent
symptom first

1. *Cessation of breathing*
2. *Eye injury*
3. *Skin contact*
4. *Shock*

Index of Products

	SYMPTOMS	INHALATION	INGESTION	SKIN	EYES
CALCIUM CHLORIDE	13	6	8	2	6
CALCIUM DICHROMATE	3	7	2	2	6
CALCIUM HYDROXIDE	20	2	3	9	3
CALCIUM HYPOCHLORITE	3	7	2	2	6
CALCIUM OXIDE	5	7	3	4	2
(Calomel) *see* MERCUROUS CHLORIDE					
(Carbolic acid) *see* PHENOL					
CARBON	14	6	10	7	7
CARBON BLACK	14	6	10	7	7
CARBON DIOXIDE	6	3	—	5	4
CARBON DIOXIDE SNOW	6	3	—	5	4
(Carbonic anhydride) *see* CARBON DIOXIDE					
CARBON MONOXIDE	6	3	—	—	—
CARBON TETRACHLORIDE	9	3	5	6	5
(Caustic lyes)	5	7	3	4	2
(Caustic potash) *see* POTASSIUM HYDROXIDE					
(Caustic soda) *see* SODIUM HYDROXIDE					
CHERRY LAUREL WATER	25	—	11	8	5
CHLORINATED LIME	3	7	2	2	6
CHLORINE	1	1	1	1	1
CHLORINE DIOXIDE	1	1	1	1	1
CHLOROACETIC ACID	1	1	1	1	1
CHLOROBENZENE	9	3	5	6	5
CHLORODIFLUOROETHANE	6	3	—	5	4
CHLORODIFLUOROMETHANE	6	3	—	5	4
CHLOROETHANES (Mono-, Di-)	9	3	5	5	4
CHLOROETHANES (Tri-, Tetra-)	9	3	5	6	5
(Chloroethylene) *see* VINYL CHLORIDE					
CHLOROFLUOROETHANES	6	3	—	5	4
CHLOROFLUOROMETHANES	6	3	—	5	4
CHLOROFORM	9	3	5	6	5
CHLOROMETHANE (Mono-)	6	3	—	5	4
CHLOROMETHANE (Di-)	6	3	5	5	4
CHLOROMETHANE (Tri-, Tetra-)	9	3	5	6	5
CHLORONAPHTHALENES	29	2	10	9	6
CHLORONITROBENZENES	11	4	7	6	3

		SYMPTOMS	INHALATION	INGESTION	SKIN	EYES
	CHLOROPENTAFLUOROETHANE	9	3	5	6	5
	CHLOROPROPANES	9	3	5	6	5
	CHLOROPROPENES	9	3	5	6	5
	(Chloropropylenes) *see* CHLOROPROPENES					
	CHLOROTRIFLUOROETHYLENE	6	3	—	5	4
	CHLOROTRIFLUOROMETHANE	6	3	—	5	4
	CHLORTHION*	23	3	5	11	9
	CHROMIC ACID	3	7	2	2	6
	CHROMIUM CHLORIDE	3	7	2	2	6
	COPPER CHLORIDE	3	7	2	2	6
	COPPER SULFATE	3	7	2	2	6
	(Corrosive sublimate) *see* MERCURIC CHLORIDE					
	CYANOGEN CHLORIDE	25	8	11	8	5
	CYCLOHEXANE	7	3	4	6	5
D	DDVP*	23	3	5	11	9
	DECANE	7	3	4	6	5
	(Decanoic alcohol) *see* DECANOL					
	DECANOL	8	3	5	6	5
	(Decyl alcohol) *see* DECANOL					
	DEMETON*	23	3	5	11	9
	DIAZINON*	23	3	5	11	9
	DIBUTYLAMINES	19	1	3	4	2
	DIBUTYLLEAD	18	5	9	6	6
	DIBUTYLTIN	22	5	9	2	6
	DICHLOROBENZENES	9	3	5	6	5
	DICHLORODIFLUOROMETHANE	6	3	—	5	4
	DICHLOROETHANES	9	3	5	5	4
	DICHLOROETHYLENES	9	3	5	6	5
	DICHLOROFLUOROMETHANE	6	3	—	5	4
	(Dichloromethane) *see* METHYLENE CHLORIDE					
	DICHLOROPROPANES	9	3	5	6	5
	DICHLOROTETRAFLUOROETHANES	9	3	5	6	5

*See Glossary of Commercial Names on page 217.

	SYMPTOMS	INHALATION	INGESTION	SKIN	EYES
DIEPOXYBUTANE	17	4	2	6	5
DIETHYLALUMINUM CHLORIDE	28	6	—	10	8
DIETHYLALUMINUM HYDRIDE	28	6	—	10	8
DIETHYLAMINE	19	1	3	4	2
DIETHYLENE GLYCOL	8	3	5	6	5
(*0,0*-Diethyl *0*-2-[ethylthio]-ethyl phosphorothioate) *see* DEMETON					
(*0,0*-Diethyl *0*-[2-isopropyl-4-methyl-6-pyrimidinyl] phosphorothioate) *see* DIAZINON					
DIETHYLLEAD	18	5	9	6	6
DIETHYLMERCURY	15	5	9	2	6
(Diethyl *para*-nitrophenyl phosphate) *see* PARA-OXON					
(*0,0*-Diethyl *0-para*-nitrophenyl phosphorothiotc) *see* PARATHION					
DIETHYLTIN	22	5	9	2	6
DIFLUOROETHANES	6	3	—	5	4
DIFLUOROETHYLENES	6	3	—	5	4
DIFLUOROMETHANE	6	3	—	5	4
DIGLYCIDYL ETHER	17	4	2	6	5
DIHEXYLTIN	22	5	9	2	6
DIIODODIETHYLTIN	22	5	9	2	6
DIISOBUTYLCARBINOL	8	3	5	6	5
DIMETHYLAMINE	19	1	3	4	2
DIMETHYLANILINE	11	4	7	6	3
(Dimethyl dichlorovinyl phosphate) *see* DDVP					
(2,6-Dimethyl-4-heptanol) *see* DIISOBUTYLCARBINOL					
(*0,0*-Dimethyl(2,2,2-trichloro-l-hydroxyethyl) phosphonate) *see* DIPTEREX					
DIMETHYLMERCURY	15	5	9	2	6
DIMETHYLTIN	22	5	9	2	6
DINITROBENZENES	11	4	7	6	3
(4,6-Dinitro-2-*sec*-butylphenol) *see* DNBP					
(4,6-Dinitro-2-*t*-butylphenol) *see* DNBP					
DINITROCRESOLS	26	4	7	6	3

*See Glossary of Commercial Names on page 217.

		SYMPTOMS	INHALATION	INGESTION	SKIN	EYES
	ETHYL NITRATE	26	4	7	6	3
	(Ethyl parathion) *see* PARATHION					
F	FERRICYANIDES (K, Na)	25	8	11	8	5
	FERROCYANIDES (K, Na)	25	8	11	8	5
	FLUORINE	2	1	1	3	1
	(Fluorocarbons) *see* FREONS					
	(Fluoroethylene) *see* VINYL FLUORIDE					
	FLUOROMETHANE	6	3	—	5	4
	FLUOSILICIC ACID	2	1	1	3	1
	(Fluothanes) *see* FREONS					
	FORMALDEHYDE	1	1	1	1	1
	(Formalin) *see* FORMALDEHYDE					
	FORMIC ACID	1	1	1	1	1
	(Formic aldehyde) *see* FORMALDEHYDE					
	FREON 11	6	3	—	5	4
	FREON 12	6	3	—	5	4
	FREON 13	6	3	—	5	4
	FREON 14	6	3	—	5	4
	FREON 21	6	3	—	5	4
	FREON 22	6	3	—	5	4
	FREON 112	9	3	5	6	5
	FREON 113	9	3	5	6	5
	FREON 114	9	3	5	6	5
	FREON 115	9	3	5	6	5
	FREON 116	6	3	—	5	4
	FREON 142b	6	3	—	5	4
	FREON 143	6	3	—	5	4
	FREON 151a	6	3	—	5	4
	FREON 152a	6	3	—	5	4
G	GASOLINE	7	3	4	6	5
	GLYCERIN	8	3	5	6	5
	GLYCIDOL	17	4	2	6	5
	GLYCIDYL ACRYLATE	17	4	2	6	5
	(Gramoxon*)	30	4	5	6	5

*See Glossary of Commercial Names on page 217.

		SYMPTOMS	INHALATION	INGESTION	SKIN	EYES
H	HEPTANE	7	3	4	6	5
	(Heptanoic alcohol) *see* HEPTANOL					
	HEPTANOL	8	3	5	6	5
	(Heptyl alcohol) *see* HEPTANOL					
	HEXACHLOROETHANE	9	3	5	6	5
	HEXAFLUOROETHANE	6	3	—	5	4
	HEXANE	7	3	4	6	5
	(Hexanoic alcohol) *see* HEXANOL					
	HEXANOL	8	3	5	6	5
	(Hexyl alcohol) *see* HEXANOL					
	HYDRIODIC ACID	1	1	1	1	1
	HYDROBROMIC ACID	1	1	1	1	1
	HYDROCHLORIC ACID	1	1	1	1	1
	HYDROCYANIC ACID	25	8	11	8	5
	HYDROFLUORIC ACID	2	1	1	3	1
	(Hydrogen arsenide) (gas) *see* ARSINE					
	(Hydrogen bromide) *see* HYDROBROMIC ACID					
	(Hydrogen chloride)	1	1	1	1	1
	(Hydrogen cyanide) *see* HYDROCYANIC ACID					
	(Hydrogen fluoride) *see* HYDROFLUORIC ACID					
	HYDROGEN PEROXIDE	1	1	1	1	1
	(Hydrogen phosphide) *see* PHOSPHINE					
	HYDROGEN SELENIDE	4	1	—	1	1
	HYDROGEN SULFIDE	4	1	—	1	1
I	IODINE	1	1	1	1	1
	IRON CHLORIDE	3	7	2	2	6
	ISOBUTYL ACETATE	8	3	5	6	5
	ISOBUTYRALDEHYDE	1	1	1	1	1
	(Isobutyric aldehyde) *see* ISOBUTYRALDEHYDE					
	ISOCYANATES	17	4	2	6	5
	ISOPESTOX*	23	3	5	11	9
	ISOPROPYL ACETATE	8	3	5	6	5

*See Glossary of Commercial Names on page 217.

		SYMPTOMS	INHALATION	INGESTION	SKIN	EYES
K	KAOLIN	14	6	10	7	7
L	LEAD (metal fumes)	24	6	2	—	6
	LEAD ACETATE	24	6	2	2	6
	LEAD ANTIMONATE	24	6	2	2	6
	LEAD ARSENATE	24	6	2	2	6
	LEAD CARBONATE	24	6	2	2	6
	LEAD CHLORIDE	24	6	2	2	6
	LEAD CHROMATE (red)	24	6	2	2	6
	LEAD CHROMATE (yellow)	24	6	2	2	6
	LEAD DIOXIDE	24	6	2	2	6
	LEAD NITRATE	24	6	2	2	6
	LEAD OLEATE	18	5	9	6	6
	LEAD OXIDE (PbO)	24	6	2	2	6
	LEAD OXIDE (red)	24	6	2	2	6
	LEAD OXYCHLORIDE	24	6	2	2	6
	LEAD PHENATE	18	5	9	6	6
	LEAD PHTHALATE	18	5	9	6	6
	LEAD STEARATE	18	5	9	6	6
	LEAD SUBACETATE	24	6	2	2	6
	LEAD SULFIDE	24	6	2	2	6
	(Lime)	5	7	3	4	2
	LITHIUM CARBONATE	20	2	3	9	3
M	MAGNESIUM CHLORIDE	27	6	—	7	6
	MAGNESIUM SULFATE	27	6	—	7	6
	MALATHION*	23	3	5	11	9
	MERCURIC CHLORIDE	16	5	2	2	6
	MERCURIC IODIDE	16	5	2	2	6
	MERCUROUS CHLORIDE	16	5	2	2	6
	MERCUROUS IODIDE	16	5	2	2	6
	MERCURY (metal)	16	5	2	2	6
	MERCURY (organic compounds)	15	5	9	2	6
	MERCURY (soluble salts)	16	5	2	2	6
	MERCURY ACETATE	16	5	2	2	6

*See Glossary of Commercial Names on page 217.

*See Glossary of Commercial Names on page 217.

		SYMPTOMS	INHALATION	INGESTION	SKIN	EYES
N	NAPHTHALENE	29	2	10	9	6
	NAPHTHYLAMINES	29	2	10	9	6
	NICKEL (fumes and dust)	17	4	2	6	5
	NICKEL CARBONYL	17	4	2	6	5
	NITRIC ACID	1	1	1	1	1
	NITROANILINES	11	4	7	6	3
	NITROBENZENE	11	4	7	6	3
	NITROFERRICYANIDES	25	8	11	8	5
	NITROGEN	6	3	—	5	4
	NITROGLYCERIN	26	4	7	6	3
	NITROPHENOLS	26	4	7	6	3
	NONANE	7	3	4	6	5
O	(Octamethyl pyrophosphoramide) *see* OMPA					
	OCTANE	7	3	4	6	5
	OMPA*	23	3	5	11	9
	ORGANOPHOSPHORUS COMPOUNDS	23	3	5	11	9
	OSMIC ACID	1	1	1	1	1
	OXALIC ACID	1	2	1	1	1
	OZONE	1	1	—	1	1
P	PARAFFINS (solid compounds)	29	2	10	—	6
	PARAOXON*	23	3	5	11	9
	PARAQUAT*	30	4	5	6	5
	PARATHION*	23	3	5	11	9
	PENTACHLOROETHANE	9	3	5	6	5
	PENTACHLOROPHENATES	26	4	7	6	3
	PENTACHLOROPHENOL	26	4	7	6	3
	PENTANE	7	3	4	6	5
	(Pentanoic alcohol) *see* PENTANOL					
	PENTANOL	8	3	5	6	5
	(Pentyl alcohol) *see* PENTANOL					
	PERACETIC ACID	1	1	1	1	1
	PERBORATES (K, Na)	3	7	2	2	6
	PERCHLORIC ACID	1	1	1	1	1

*See Glossary of Commercial Names on page 217.

	SYMPTOMS	INHALATION	INGESTION	SKIN	EYES
(Perchloroethylene) *see* TETRACHLOROETHYLENE					
(Perfluoroethylene) *see* TETRAFLUOROETHYLENE					
(Petrol) *see* GASOLINE					
PETROLEUM ETHERS	7	3	4	6	5
PHENOL	1	1	1	1	1
PHENYLHYDRAZINE	11	4	7	6	3
PHENYLHYDROXYLAMINE	11	4	7	6	3
PHENYLMERCURIC ACETATE	15	5	9	2	6
PHENYLMERCURY	15	5	9	2	6
PHENYLMERCURY OLEATE	15	5	9	2	6
PHENYLNAPHTHYLAMINES	29	2	10	9	6
PHOSDRIN*	23	3	5	11	9
PHOSGENE	1	1	—	1	1
PHOSPHINE	21	1	—	1	1
PHOSPHORIC ACID	1	1	1	1	1
PHOSPHORIC ESTERS	23	3	5	11	9
PHOSPHORUS CHLORIDES	21	1	1	1	1
PHOSPHORUS PENTACHLORIDE	21	1	1	1	1
PHOSPHORUS TRICHLORIDE	21	1	1	1	1
PHTHALIC ANHYDRIDE	3	7	2	2	6
POLY(VINYL CHLORIDE)	14	6	10	7	7
POTASSIUM (metal)	5	7	3	4	2
POTASSIUM BORATE	3	7	2	2	6
POTASSIUM CARBONATE	20	2	3	9	3
POTASSIUM CHLORATE	12	2	8	2	6
POTASSIUM CHLORIDE	13	6	8	2	6
POTASSIUM CHLORITE	1	1	1	1	1
POTASSIUM CHROMATE	3	7	2	2	6
POTASSIUM CYANIDE	25	8	11	8	5
POTASSIUM DICHROMATE	3	7	2	2	6
POTASSIUM FLUORIDE	2	1	1	3	1
POTASSIUM FLUOSILICATE	2	7	1	3	1
POTASSIUM HYDROXIDE	5	7	3	4	2

*See Glossary of Commercial Names on page 217.

*See Glossary of Commercial Names on page 217.

		SYMPTOMS	INHALATION	INGESTION	SKIN	EYES
	SODIUM FLUORIDE	2	1	1	3	1
	SODIUM FLUOSILICATE	2	7	1	3	1
	SODIUM HYDROXIDE	5	7	3	4	2
	SODIUM HYPOCHLORITE	3	7	2	2	6
	SODIUM OXIDE	5	7	3	4	2
	SODIUM PERCHLORATE	12	2	8	2	6
	SODIUM PEROXIDE	5	7	3	4	2
	(Sodium phosphate-trisodium) *see* TRISODIUM PHOSPHATE					
	SODIUM SILICATE	20	2	3	9	3
	SODIUM SULFATE	27	6	—	7	6
	SODIUM THIOCYANATE	27	6	—	8	5
	SODIUM THIOSULFATE	27	6	—	7	6
	STYRENE	17	4	2	6	5
	SULFOTEPP*	23	3	5	11	9
	SULFUR DIOXIDE	1	1	1	1	1
	SULFURIC ACID	1	1	1	1	1
	(Sulfuric ether) *see* ETHYL ETHER					
	SULFUROUS ACID	1	1	1	1	1
	SULFUR TRIOXIDE	1	1	1	1	1
	(Systox) *see* DEMETON					
T	TALC	14	6	10	7	7
	TEPP*	23	3	5	11	9
	TETRABUTYLTIN	22	5	9	2	6
	TETRACHLORODIFLUOROETHANES	9	3	5	6	5
	TETRACHLOROETHANES	9	3	5	6	5
	TETRACHLOROETHYLENE	9	3	5	6	5
	(Tetrachloromethane) *see* CARBON TETRACHLORIDE					
	(Tetraethyl dithiopyrophosphate) *see* SULFOTEPP					
	TETRAETHYLLEAD	18	5	9	6	6
	(Tetraethyl pyrophosphate) *see* TEPP					
	TETRAETHYLTIN	22	5	9	2	6

*See Glossary of Commercial Names on page 217.

	SYMPTOMS	INHALATION	INGESTION	SKIN	EYES
TETRAFLUOROETHYLENE	6	3	—	5	4
TETRAFLUOROMETHANE	6	3	—	5	4
TETRAISOALKYLTINS	22	5	9	2	6
TETRAMETHYLLEAD	18	5	9	6	6
TETRAPENTYLTIN	22	5	9	2	6
TETRAPROPYLTIN	22	5	9	2	6
THIOCYANATES	27	6	11	8	5
TIN (organic compounds)	22	5	9	2	6
TITANIUM (dust)	14	6	10	7	7
TITANIUM CHLORIDES (Tri, Tetra-)	3	7	2	2	6
TITANIUM OXIDE	14	6	10	7	7
TOLUENE	7	3	4	6	5
TOLUIDINES	11	4	7	6	3
TRIBUTYLLEAD	18	5	9	6	6
TRIBUTYLTIN	22	5	9	2	6
TRICHLOROACETIC ACID	1	1	1	1	1
TRICHLOROETHANES	9	3	5	6	5
TRICHLOROETHYLENE	9	3	5	6	5
TRICHLOROFLUOROMETHANE	6	3	—	5	4
(Trichloromethane) *see* CHLOROFORM					
TRICHLOROTRIFLUOROETHANES	9	3	5	6	5
TRIETHYLALUMINUM	28	6	—	10	8
TRIETHYLAMINE	19	1	3	4	2
TRIETHYLENE GLYCOL	8	3	5	6	5
TRIETHYLLEAD	18	5	9	6	6
TRIETHYLTIN	22	5	9	2	6
TRIFLUOROETHANES	6	3	—	5	4
TRIFLUOROMETHANE	6	3	—	5	4
TRIISOBUTYLALUMINUM	28	6	—	10	8
TRIMETHYLALUMINUM	28	6	—	10	8
TRIMETHYLAMINE	19	1	3	4	2
TRIMETHYLLEAD	18	5	9	6	6
TRIMETHYLTIN	22	5	9	2	6
TRINITROBENZENE	11	4	7	6	3
TRIPHENYLTIN	22	5	9	2	6
TRIPROPYLTIN	22	5	9	2	6
TRISODIUM PHOSPHATE (Na_3PO_4)	20	2	3	9	3

		SYMPTOMS	INHALATION	INGESTION	SKIN	EYES
	TRITHION*	23	3	5	11	9
	TUNGSTEN CARBIDE	14	6	10	7	7
V	VINYL ACETATE	8	3	5	6	5
	VINYL CHLORIDE	9	3	5	5	4
	VINYL FLUORIDE	6	3	—	5	4
	VINYLIDENE CHLORIDE	9	3	5	5	4
	VINYLIDENE FLUORIDE	6	3	—	5	4
W	WHITE SPIRIT	7	3	4	6	5
X	XYLENES	7	3	4	6	5
	XYLIDINES	11	4	7	6	3
Z	ZINC CHLORIDE	3	7	2	2	6

*See Glossary of Commercial Names on page 217.

Description of Symptoms of Poisoning

1

ACETALDEHYDE
ACETIC ACID
ACETIC ANHYDRIDE
ACROLEIN
BROMINE
BUTYRALDEHYDE
CHLORINE
CHLORINE DIOXIDE
CHLOROACETIC ACID
ETHYL CHLOROFORMATE
FORMALDEHYDE
FORMIC ACID
HYDRIODIC ACID
HYDROBROMIC ACID
HYDROCHLORIC ACID
(Hydrogen chloride)
HYDROGEN PEROXIDE
IODINE
ISOBUTYRALDEHYDE
METHYL CHLOROFORMATE
NITRIC ACID
OSMIC ACID
OXALIC ACID
OZONE
PERACETIC ACID
PERCHLORIC ACID
PHENOL
PHOSGENE
PHOSPHORIC ACID
POTASSIUM CHLORITE
PROPIONALDEHYDE
SODIUM CHLORITE
SULFUR DIOXIDE
SULFURIC ACID
SULFUROUS ACID
SULFUR TRIOXIDE
TRICHLOROACETIC ACID

The above caustic (corrosive) substances all give off irritating vapors or fumes as soon as they come into contact with mucous membranes or moist skin.

Chlorites give off CHLORINE DIOXIDE as soon as they come into contact with dilute acid.

The concentration and composition of these products will determine seriousness of injury.

I. INHALATION

A. Symptoms of acute poisoning

1. Irritation of mucous membranes (nose, mouth, eyes, throat)
2. Watering of eyes, nasal discharge, sneezing, coughing (head cold)
3. Thoracic oppression and distress
4. Difficulty in breathing

5. Rapid breathing
6. Fits of coughing
7. Headache
8. BLUISH face and lips
9. Salivation
10. Giddiness
11. Nausea
12. Muscular weakness
13. Ulceration of mucous membranes (nose)
14. Chemical bronchitis
15. Acute pulmonary edema
16. Secondary chemical pneumonia
17. Death

(14–16: diagnosis can only be made by a physician)

B. First aid: see **yellow** pages, section **1**
see **yellow** pages, section **2** (OXALIC ACID only)

II. INGESTION

A. Symptoms of acute poisoning

1. Irritation and burning sensation of lips, mouth, and throat
2. Pain in swallowing
3. Abundant salivation
4. Ulceration of the mucous membranes and color change of the tongue (GRAY with HYDROCHLORIC ACID, YELLOW with NITRIC ACID, WHITE to BLACK with SULFURIC ACID, WHITE with HYDROGEN PEROXIDE, OXALIC ACID, and PHENOL)
5. Intense thirst

6. Edema of the glottis (diagnosis can only be made by a physician)
7. Burning sensation at the esophagus, back of throat, and stomach
8. Painful abdominal cramps
9. Nausea and vomiting, occasionally of blood (digestive hemorrhage)
10. Difficulty in breathing
11. Risk of perforation of the stomach
12. State of shock
    - weak and rapid pulse
    - cold sweat—pale complexion
    - tendency to fainting
    - cold hands and feet
13. Convulsions
14. Coma
15. Death

B. First aid: see **green** pages, section **1**

III. SKIN CONTACT

PHENOL, which penetrates healthy skin, may cause general poisoning resulting in death.

Vapors are less irritating to the skin than solutions, where the concentration and the length of contact determine the gravity of the symptoms.

In an accident where volatile products come in contact with the skin, poisoning by inhalation will frequently occur.

A. Immediate symptoms

1. Smarting
2. Burning sensation

3. Inflammation
4. Burns that may be very painful and become WHITE (in the case of HYDROCHLORIC ACID, HYDROGEN PEROXIDE, and PHENOL) or YELLOW (in the case of NITRIC ACID)
5. Painful blisters
6. Profound damage to tissues (painless in the case of PHENOL)
7. Shock can occur as a result of pain
   - weak and rapid pulse
   - cold sweat—pale complexion
   - tendency to fainting
   - cold hands and feet
8. Lingering death (PHENOL only)

B. First aid: see **pink** pages, section **1**

IV. SPLASHING OF LIQUID IN OR CONTACT OF VAPOR WITH EYES

In an accident caused by volatile products, poisoning by inhalation will frequently occur.

A. Immediate symptoms

1. Stinging or burning sensation
2. Watering of eyes
3. Conjunctivitis (inflammation of eyes)
4. Burning sensation in eyelids and eyes, with ulceration of the tissues
5. Yellow eyes (NITRIC ACID only)
6. Opaqueness of the cornea
7. Loss of sight

B. First aid: see **blue** pages, section **1**

2

FLUORINE
FLUOSILICIC ACID
HYDROFLUORIC ACID
POTASSIUM FLUORIDE
POTASSIUM FLUOSILICATE
SODIUM FLUORIDE
SODIUM FLUOSILICATE

HYDROFLUORIC ACID is a strong acid with a highly caustic and corrosive effect on organic tissue. The resulting burns often do not become painful until several hours later. Fluosilicates are less irritating but are toxic to liver and kidneys.

I. INHALATION

A. Symptoms of acute poisoning

1. Irritation of mucous membranes (nose, eyes, mouth, throat)
2. Watering of eyes
3. Salivation
4. Fits of coughing
5. Ulceration of mucous membranes (nose and throat)
6. Pain in throat
7. Thoracic congestion
8. Difficulty in breathing
9. Bronchitis
10. Headache
11. Fatigue
12. Giddiness
13. Nausea
14. Stomach pains
15. Pale or BLUISH face

16. State of shock
    - weak and rapid pulse
    - cold sweat—pale complexion
    - tendency to fainting
    - cold hands and feet
17. Chemical pneumonia (diagnosis can only be made by a physician)
18. Coma
19. Acute pulmonary edema (diagnosis can only be made by a physician)
20. Death

B. First aid: see **yellow** pages, section **1**
see **yellow** pages, section **7** (Fluosilicates only)

II. INGESTION

A. Symptoms of acute poisoning

1. Irritation and painful burning sensation of lips, mouth, and throat
2. Ulceration of mucous membranes
3. Pain in swallowing
4. Edema of the glottis (diagnosis can only be made by a physician)
5. Intense thirst
6. Violent burning sensation in the esophagus and stomach
7. Painful stomach cramps with distension of stomach
8. Difficulty in breathing
9. Muscular fatigue and general weakness
10. Coughing
11. Acute pulmonary edema
12. Perforation of stomach

(11–12: diagnosis can only be made by a physician)

13. Nausea and vomiting, occasionally of blood (digestive hemorrhage)
14. Pale or BLUISH face
15. State of shock
    - weak and rapid pulse
    - cold sweat—pale complexion
    - tendency to fainting
    - cold hands and feet
16. Convulsions
17. Coma
18. Death

B. First aid: see **green** pages, section **1**

III. SKIN CONTACT

A. Immediate symptoms

1. Burning sensation and inflammation
2. Irreparable damage to skin, which gradually turns white and becomes very painful
3. Blisters
4. Profound damage to the tissues
5. Shock may occur as a result of pain
    - weak and rapid pulse
    - cold sweat—pale complexion
    - tendency to fainting
    - cold hands and feet

B. First aid: see **pink** pages, section **3**

IV. SPLASHING OF LIQUID IN OR CONTACT OF VAPOR WITH EYES

A. Immediate symptoms

1. Intense stinging and burning sensation
2. Watering of eyes
3. Conjunctivitis (inflammation of eyes)
4. Burning sensation in eyelids and eyes, with ulceration of the tissues
5. Irreparable damage to cornea
6. Loss of vision

B. First aid: see **blue** pages, section **1**

ALKALI DICHROMATES (Ca, K, Na)
ALKALI *META*-BORATES (K, Na)
ALUMINUM CHLORIDE
(Aluminum trichloride)
BORIC ACID
CALCIUM DICHROMATE
CALCIUM HYPOCHLORITE
CHLORINATED LIME
CHROMIC ACID
CHROMIUM CHLORIDE
COPPER CHLORIDE
COPPER SULFATE
IRON CHLORIDE
PERBORATES (K, Na)
PHTHALIC ANHYDRIDE
POTASSIUM BORATE
POTASSIUM CHROMATE
POTASSIUM DICHROMATE
SODIUM BORATE
SODIUM CHROMATE
SODIUM DICHROMATE
SODIUM HYPOCHLORITE
TITANIUM CHLORIDES
(Tri-, Tetra-)
ZINC CHLORIDE

In aqueous solution, these substances are all irritating to mucous membranes of the digestive system and eyes, in addition to the specific toxicity of their cations.

TITANIUM TETRACHLORIDE hydrolyzes rapidly and produces HYDROGEN CHLORIDE (see **white** pages, section **1**, p. 31).

I. INHALATION OF DUST

A. Symptoms of very acute poisoning

1. Irritation of nose and eyes
2. Fits of coughing, sometimes violent
3. Difficulty in breathing
4. BLUISH face and lips
5. Risk of pulmonary edema

B. Symptoms of acute poisoning

1. Irritation of nose and eyes

2. Tingling and burning sensation in respiratory tract
3. Sneezing

C. First aid: see **yellow** pages, section **7**

II. INGESTION

A. Symptoms of acute poisoning

1. Burning sensation in mouth and throat
2. Salivation
3. Burning sensation in stomach
4. Stomach cramps
5. Nausea and vomiting, occasionally of blood (digestive hemorrhage)
6. General weakness, dizziness
7. Diarrhea, possibly blood-stained
8. State of shock
    - weak and rapid pulse
    - cold sweat—pale complexion
    - tendency to fainting
    - cold hands and feet
9. Possible convulsions
10. Risk of paralysis (MAGNESIUM CHLORIDE only)
11. Coma
12. Death

B. First aid: see **green** pages, section **2**

III. CONTACT WITH MOIST SKIN

A. Immediate symptoms

1. Itching
2. Irritation and burning sensation
3. Inflammation
4. Ulceration and possibly profound necrosis (destruction of tissue)

B. First aid: see **pink** pages, section **2**

IV. SPLASHING IN EYES

A. Immediate symptoms

1. Stinging and burning sensation
2. Watering of eyes
3. Inflammation of conjunctivas
4. Risk of serious lesions

B. First aid: see **blue** pages, section **6**

HYDROGEN SELENIDE HYDROGEN SULFIDE

Colorless gases with a strong smell of garlic or rotten eggs, highly toxic and irritating to mucous membranes of the respiratory system and eyes.

I. INHALATION

A. Symptoms of very acute poisoning

1. Sudden loss of consciousness
2. Breathing stops abruptly
3. Death follows quickly

B. Symptoms of acute poisoning

1. Irritation of nose, throat, and eyes
2. Sneezing
3. Headache
4. Excitability
5. Dizziness, staggering
6. Nausea and vomiting
7. Breathing difficulties
8. Pale complexion
9. Dry cough
10. Cold sweat
11. Diarrhea
12. Muscular weakness
13. Drowsiness
14. Chemical bronchitis (diagnosis can only be made by a physician)
15. Risk of pulmonary edema

16. Death

B. First aid: see **yellow** pages, section **1**

II. INGESTION

No risk

III. SKIN CONTACT

The vapors cause no adverse symptoms on skin, even in toxic concentrations.

The solutions may be irritating.

A. Immediate symptoms

1. Slight irritation
2. Painful inflammation
3. Possible discoloration

B. First aid: see **pink** pages, section **1**

IV. CONTACT OF VAPOR WITH EYES

A. Immediate symptoms

1. Irritation
2. Watering of eyes
3. Inflammation of conjunctivas
4. Risk of serious lesions

B. First aid: see **blue** pages, section **1**

CALCIUM CARBIDE*
CALCIUM OXIDE
(Caustic lyes)
(Lime)
POTASSIUM (metal)
POTASSIUM HYDROXIDE
POTASSIUM OXIDE
SODIUM (metal)
SODIUM HYDROXIDE
SODIUM OXIDE
SODIUM PEROXIDE

These substances are particularly caustic (corrosive) in contact with mucous membranes and moist skin. They all give off heat when dissolved in water. This increases their corrosiveness since they are capable of dissolving living tissue.

*When CALCIUM CARBIDE comes into contact with moist skin, it decomposes into CALCIUM OXIDE, hydroxide, and ACETYLENE, while PHOSPHINE and ARSINE are formed from impurities (see **white** pages, section **21**, page 93).

I. INHALATION OF DUST

A. Symptoms of very acute poisoning

1. Irritation of nose, eyes, and throat
2. Burning sensation in nose and throat
3. Difficulty in breathing
4. Fits of coughing
5. Chemical, secondary bronchitis or pneumonia (diagnosis can only be made by a physician)
6. Risk of acute pulmonary edema

B. Symptoms of acute poisoning

1. Irritation of nose and eyes
2. Sneezing

3. Tingling sensation in nose and throat
4. Cough
5. Risk of chemical bronchitis

C. First aid: see **yellow** pages, section 7

II. INGESTION

A. Symptoms of acute poisoning

1. Immediate, intense burning sensation in mouth, throat, and stomach
2. Immediate effect on buccal (cheeks and mouth cavity) membranes, which become white
3. Intense pain in swallowing
4. Edema of the glottis (diagnosis can only be made by a physician)
5. Strong salivation, which increases the pain
6. Vomiting; vomit is brown and contains pieces of mucous membrane of the stomach (digestive hemorrhage)
7. Stomach cramps
8. Rapid breathing
9. State of shock
   - weak and rapid pulse
   - cold sweat—pale complexion
   - tendency to fainting
   - cold hands and feet
10. Diarrhea, possibly blood-stained
11. Risk of perforation of stomach
12. Loss of consciousness

13. Death

B. First aid: see **green** pages, section **3**

III. SKIN CONTACT

A. Immediate symptoms

1. Itching and tingling sensation
2. Painful sensation
3. Painful ulceration
4. Profound, irreparable damage of tissues
5. State of shock
   - weak and rapid pulse
   - cold sweat—pale complexion
   - tendency to fainting
   - cold hands and feet

B. First aid: see **pink** pages, section **4**

IV. SPLASHING IN EYES

A. Immediate or delayed symptoms

1. Highly painful, instantaneous irritation of eyes and eyelids
2. Intense watering of eyes
3. Victim keeps eyelids tightly closed
4. Burns and irreparable damage of mucous membranes
5. Ulceration of eyes

6. Perforation of eyes
7. Loss of eyes

NOTE: If only one eye is splashed and first aid is not given **immediately**, the other eye may be lost as well, even if **the substance has not come into contact with it!**

B. First aid: see **blue** pages, section **2**

ACETYLENE (pure material)*
ALKANES (gases) (C_1 to C_4)
BUTADIENE
BUTANE
CARBON DIOXIDE
CARBON DIOXIDE SNOW
CARBON MONOXIDE
CHLORODIFLUOROETHANE
CHLORODIFLUOROMETHANE
CHLOROFLUOROETHANES
CHLOROFLUOROMETHANES
CHLOROMETHANE (Mono-, Di-)
CHLOROTRIFLUOROETHYLENE
CHLOROTRIFLUOROMETHANE
DICHLORODIFLUOROMETHANE
DICHLOROFLUOROMETHANE
DIFLUOROETHANES
DIFLUOROETHYLENES
DIFLUOROMETHANE
ETHANE
ETHYLENE
ETHYL ETHER
ETHYL FLUORIDE
FLUOROMETHANE
FREON 11, 12, 13, 14, 21, 22, 116, 142b, 143, 151a, 152a
HEXAFLUOROETHANE
METHANE
METHYL CHLORIDE
METHYLENE CHLORIDE
METHYLENE FLUORIDE
NITROGEN
PROPANE
PROPYLENE
TETRAFLUOROETHYLENE
TETRAFLUOROMETHANE
TRICHLOROFLUOROMETHANE
TRIFLUOROETHANES
TRIFLUOROMETHANE
VINYL FLUORIDE
VINYLIDENE FLUORIDE

These substances are gaseous at room temperature, practically nonirritating and, with the exception of CARBON MONOXIDE, nontoxic as such. However, in high concentrations they all cause **asphyxia** by displacing oxygen. METHYL CHLORIDE and METHYLENE CHLORIDE cause lesions in the cornea due to inflammation.

*In the case of technical grade acetylene, highly toxic impurities such as ARSINE and PHOSPHINE (see **white** pages, section **21**, page 93) should be taken into account.

I. INHALATION

A. Symptoms following severe exposure

ASPHYXIA

1. Need for fresh air

2. Rapid, occasionally irregular, breathing
3. Headache
4. Fatigue
5. Mental confusion
6. Nausea and vomiting
7. Giddiness
8. Exhaustion
9. Loss of consciousness
10. Convulsions
11. Death

B. First aid: see **yellow** pages, section **3**

II. INGESTION

Practically no risk, except for ETHYL ETHER

A. Symptoms of severe ether poisoning

1. Breath has ethereal smell
2. Rapid intoxication
3. Drowsiness

B. First aid: see **green** pages, section **4**

III. SKIN CONTACT

The gaseous substances have no effect on the skin.

Splashes of the liquid substances that have a low boiling point may "freeze" the skin.

A. Immediate symptoms

1. Feeling of intense cold
2. Insensitivity to pain
3. Congestion of blood vessels, rapidly becoming painful (freezing)

B. First aid: see **pink** pages, section **5**

IV. SPLASHING OF LIQUID IN EYES

The vapors have no serious irritating effect on the eyes.

When liquids that have a low boiling point are splashed in the eyes, they may cause severe "freezing."

A. Immediate or delayed symptoms

1. Stinging pain
2. Watering of eyes
3. Inflammation of conjunctivas
4. Cloudiness to opaqueness of eyes

B. First aid: see **blue** pages, section **4**

7

BENZENE
CYCLOHEXANE
DECANE
GASOLINE
HEPTANE
HEXANE
NONANE
OCTANE
PENTANE
PETROLEUM ETHERS
TOLUENE
WHITE SPIRIT
XYLENES

These substances do not appear to be toxic as such. However, their vapors are occasionally irritating to mucous membranes of the respiratory system and eyes and, in very high concentrations, they are **narcotic**.

I. INHALATION

A. Symptoms of acute poisoning

a. by vapors

1. Rapid breathing
2. Excitability, with intoxication and mental confusion
3. Staggering
4. Headache
5. Fatigue
6. Nausea with vomiting
7. Dizziness
8. Drowsiness
9. Narcosis (stupor and unconsciousness)
10. Loss of consciousness
11. Convulsions
12. Coma and death

b. by mist or fine droplets

1. Coughing
2. Difficulty in breathing
3. BLUISH face and lips
4. Nausea and vomiting
5. Fatigue
6. Bronchitis and fever
7. Chemical pneumonia
8. Acute pulmonary edema

(7–8: diagnosis can only be made by a physician)

B. First aid: see **yellow** pages, section **3**

II. INGESTION

A. Symptoms of acute poisoning

1. Slight gastro-intestinal irritation
2. Dizziness
3. Fatigue
4. Loss of consciousness
5. Coma and death

If the subject recovers, there is a risk of

6. Coughing
7. Bronchitis and fever
8. Pneumonia

B. First aid: see **green** pages, section **4**

III. SKIN CONTACT

These gaseous substances have no effect on the skin. In liquid form, they remove oils from the skin, which eventually leads to

A. Immediate or delayed symptoms

1. Dryness
2. Cracks causing irritation

B. First aid: see **pink** pages, section **6**

IV. SPLASHING OF LIQUID IN OR CONTACT OF VAPOR WITH EYES

The vapors of these substances are only slightly irritating to the eyes. Liquids are strongly irritating to the eyes and to mucous membranes.

A. Immediate symptoms

1. Stinging sensation
2. Watering of eyes
3. Inflammation of the conjunctivas

B. First aid: see **blue** pages, section **5**

8

ACETONE
ALIPHATIC ALCOHOLS
AMYL ACETATE
BUTANOL
BUTYL ACETATE
DECANOL
DIETHYLENE GLYCOL
DIISOBUTYLCARBINOL
ETHYL ACETATE
ETHYL ALCOHOL
ETHYLENE GLYCOL
ETHYLHEXYL ACETATE
GLYCERIN
HEPTANOL
HEXANOL
ISOBUTYL ACETATE
ISOPROPYL ACETATE
METHYL ACETATE
METHYL ALCOHOL
PENTANOL
PROPYL ACETATE
PROPYL ALCOHOLS
PROPYLENE GLYCOL
TRIETHYLENE GLYCOL
VINYL ACETATE

These liquids are more or less volatile and, in high concentrations, cause depression of the brain and nervous system and damage to the liver.

GLYCERIN is only slightly volatile and reputed to be nontoxic.

I. INHALATION

A. Symptoms of acute poisoning

1. Slight irritation of nose and eyes
2. Head feels hot and face is flushed
3. Excitability and talkativeness
4. Intoxication
5. Staggering and lack of coordination
6. Headache
7. Mental confusion and visual disturbance
8. Tiredness
9. Nausea and vomiting
10. Paleness of complexion

11. Dizziness
12. Eyes are sensitive to and painful in direct light (METHYL ALCOHOL only)
13. Drowsiness
14. Stupor
15. Loss of consciousness
16. Coma and death

NOTE: METHYL ALCOHOL can seriously impair vision and may cause blindness.

B. First aid: see **yellow** pages, section **3**

II. INGESTION

A. Symptoms of acute poisoning

1. Gastro-intestinal irritation
2. Followed by symptoms described in I. INHALATION

NOTE: METHYL ALCOHOL can seriously impair vision and may cause blindness. Glycol derivatives are toxic to the kidneys.

B. First aid: see **green** pages, section **5**

III. SKIN CONTACT

A. Immediate symptoms

- Highly volatile products (METHYL ALCOHOL and ACETONE) produce a feeling of cold.

- Alcohols, acetates, and ACETONE remove oils from the skin, which becomes dry and eventually develops cracks or dermatitis.
- Glycol derivatives have little effect on healthy skin.

NOTE: METHYL ALCOHOL, which can be absorbed by the skin, causes
- headache
- fatigue
- reduction of visual acuity

B. First aid: see **pink** pages, section **6**

IV. SPLASHING IN EYES

A. Immediate symptoms

1. Vapors are slightly uncomfortable; splashes are irritating
2. Irritation with painful burning or stinging sensation
3. Watering of eyes
4. Inflammation of the conjunctivas
5. Eyes are sensitive to and painful in the light

B. First aid: see **blue** pages, section **5**

CARBON TETRACHLORIDE
CHLOROBENZENE
CHLOROETHANES
(Mono-, Di-, Tri-, Tetra-)
CHLOROFORM
CHLOROMETHANES
(Tri-, Tetra-)
CHLOROPENTAFLUORO-ETHANE
CHLOROPROPANES
CHLOROPROPENES
DICHLOROBENZENES
DICHLOROETHANES
DICHLOROETHYLENES
DICHLOROPROPANES
DICHLOROTETRAFLUORO-ETHANES
FREON 112, 113, 114, 115
HEXACHLOROETHANE
(Methylchloroform)
PENTACHLOROETHANE
TETRACHLORODIFLUORO-ETHANES
TETRACHLOROETHANES
TETRACHLOROETHYLENE
TRICHLOROETHANES
TRICHLOROETHYLENE
TRICHLOROTRIFLUORO-ETHANES
VINYL CHLORIDE
VINYLIDENE CHLORIDE

The chlorinated and chlorofluorinated solvents are colorless, volatile gases or liquids that smell of chloroform. They are, in varying degrees, toxic to the nervous system, liver, and kidneys. They remove oils from skin, which eventually becomes dry and cracked.

The fluorinated solvents have little irritating or toxic effect on the nervous system.

I. INHALATION

A. Symptoms of acute poisoning

1. Irritation of eyes, nose, and throat (not in the case of METHYL CHLORIDE)
2. Overexcitement
3. Headache
4. Intoxication (staggering, loss of equilibrium)
5. Loss of consciousness
6. Narcosis (deep unconsciousness)

7. State of shock
   - weak and rapid pulse
   - cold sweat—pale complexion
   - tendency to fainting
   - cold hands and feet
8. Coma
9. Death as a result of cardiac or respiratory failure

NOTE: There is risk of acute pulmonary edema if the victim recovers.

B. Symptoms of relatively acute poisoning

1. Headache
2. Fatigue, weariness
3. Nausea, vomiting
4. Dizziness
5. Stupor
6. Drowsiness
7. Disturbed vision
8. Coughing
9. Narcosis (deep unconsciousness)

C. First aid: see **yellow** pages, section **3**

II. INGESTION

(Except for chlorinated solvents with low boiling points.)

A. Symptoms of acute poisoning

CHARACTERISTIC SYMPTOM: breath smells of chloroform

1. Irritation of lips and mouth
2. Gastro-intestinal irritation
3. Nausea, vomiting
4. Diarrhea, possibly blood-stained
5. Drowsiness
6. Loss of consciousness
7. Narcosis (deep unconsciousness)
8. State of shock
   - weak and rapid pulse
   - cold sweat—pale complexion
   - tendency to fainting
   - cold hands and feet
9. Risk of acute pulmonary edema

B. First aid: see **green** pages, section **5**

III. SKIN CONTACT

Chlorinated solvents absorbed through healthy skin may cause symptoms described under I. INHALATION, B.

A. Immediate and delayed symptoms

1. Dry skin
2. Freezing
3. Inflammation
4. Blisters that later become painful

B. First aid: see **pink** pages, section **6**
or **pink** pages, section **5**

IV. SPLASHING OF LIQUID IN OR CONTACT OF VAPOR WITH EYES

A. Immediate symptoms caused by vapors

1. Irritation of eyes
2. Watering of eyes
3. Occasionally inflammation of conjunctivas

B. Immediate symptoms when liquid is splashed in eyes

1. Burning sensation
2. Watering of eyes
3. Inflammation of conjunctivas
4. Lesions in cornea due to inflammation (VINYL CHLORIDE)

C. First aid: see **blue** pages, section **5**
or **blue** pages, section **4**

BARIUM (soluble salts)
BARIUM ACETATE
BARIUM CARBONATE
BARIUM CHLORIDE
BARIUM FLUORIDE
BARIUM HYDROXIDE
BARIUM NITRATE
BARIUM OXIDE
BARIUM SULFIDE

NOTE: Only BARIUM SULFATE is insoluble and nontoxic.

All the soluble barium compounds have a toxic effect on the nervous system and circulation and may lead to death in the course of a few hours. Soluble barium compounds occur as crystals and have a disagreeable, styptic taste.

I. INHALATION

Soluble barium compounds in the form of dust may be absorbed by nasal mucous membranes and cause a moderate degree of poisoning.

A. Symptoms of acute poisoning

1. Irritation of nose and eyes (BARIUM FLUORIDE, BARIUM HYDROXIDE, and BARIUM OXIDE)
2. Muscular fibrillation
3. Tendency to fatigue
4. Cold sweat

B. First aid: see **yellow** pages, section **2**

II. INGESTION

A. Symptoms of acute poisoning

1. Disagreeable taste
2. Muscular contractions
3. Nausea and vomiting
4. Stomach pains and diarrhea
5. Anxiety
6. Convulsions
7. BLUISH face and lips

8. State of shock
   - weak and rapid pulse
   - cold sweat—pale complexion
   - tendency to fainting
   - cold hands and feet
9. Paralysis of lower limbs, spreading to upper limbs
10. Difficulty in breathing
11. Cyanosis and death by fainting and partial or complete temporary respiratory failure or respiratory paralysis

B. First aid: see **green** pages, section **6**

III. SKIN CONTACT

BARIUM FLUORIDE, BARIUM OXIDE, and soluble salts are irritating to the skin.

1. Irritation of skin and mucous membranes
2. Prolonged contact of dusts with moist skin causes
   - ulcerations
   - necrosis (destruction of tissue) (BARIUM FLUORIDE only)

First aid: see **pink** pages, section **2**

IV. SPLASHING IN EYES

A. Immediate symptoms

1. Mechanical and chemical irritation
2. Watering of eyes
3. Inflammation of conjunctivas (BARIUM FLUORIDE, BARIUM OXIDE, and BARIUM HYDROXIDE)
4. Burning sensation

B. First aid: see **blue** pages, section **6**

ANILINE
CHLORONITROBENZENES
DIMETHYLANILINE
DINITROBENZENES
NITROANILINES
NITROBENZENES
PHENYLHYDRAZINE
PHENYLHYDROXYLAMINE
TOLUIDINES
TRINITROBENZENE
XYLIDINES

These substances are toxic to the blood and prevent hemoglobin from carrying oxygen.

I. INHALATION

A. Symptoms of acute poisoning

1. Face, lips, and hands are DEEP BLUE
2. Headache
3. Rapid and difficult breathing
4. Dizziness
5. Mental confusion
6. General weakness
7. Convulsions
8. Coma
9. Death

B. First aid: see **yellow** pages, section **4**

II. INGESTION

A. Symptoms of acute poisoning

See I. INHALATION

1. Irritation of mouth and stomach

2. Stomach cramps and diarrhea

B. First aid: see **green** pages, section **7**

III. SKIN CONTACT

Those substances that are fat-soluble can be absorbed by healthy skin and cause the same symptoms as described under I. INHALATION.

A. Additional immediate symptoms

1. Irritation
2. Small vesicles
3. Dermatitis
4. Ulceration and necrosis (destruction of tissue)

B. First aid: see **pink** pages, section **6**

IV. SPLASHING IN EYES

A. Immediate symptoms

1. Irritation
2. Inflammation of conjunctivas
3. Photophobia (abnormal intolerance of light)
4. Severe lesions

B. First aid: see **blue** pages, section **3**

AMMONIUM CHLORATE
AMMONIUM PERCHLORATE
POTASSIUM CHLORATE
POTASSIUM PERCHLORATE
SODIUM CHLORATE
SODIUM PERCHLORATE

These substances come in the form of white, highly reactive crystals.

The perchlorates, and the chlorates even more so, are toxic to the blood. They prevent hemoglobin from carrying oxygen. After 1 to 3 days, they also cause serious lesions in the liver and kidneys that may result in death.

I. INHALATION

There is little risk of poisoning because the serious risk of fire requires strict safety measures dealing with the formation of dust.

A. Symptoms of acute poisoning

1. Irritation of nose and eyes
2. Sneezing
3. Small nasal ulcerations

B. First aid: see **yellow** pages, section **2**

II. INGESTION

A. Symptoms of acute poisoning

1. Stomach pains
2. Nausea and vomiting
3. Diarrhea
4. BLUISH face and hands
5. Rapid breathing
6. Dizziness

7. Mental confusion
8. General weakness
9. Coma
10. Death

B. First aid: see **green** pages, section **8**

III. SKIN CONTACT

NOTE: Clothes that have been impregnated with chlorate or perchlorate solution may, once dry, burst spontaneously into flames; they may also burn as a result of simple friction or contact with a spark or hot cigarette ash.

Clothes that have simply been dried must not be returned to the victim. It is essential that they be washed with plenty of water.

A. Immediate symptoms

1. Slight irritation
2. Inflammation
3. Ulcerations may follow later

B. First aid: see **pink** pages, section **2**

IV. SPLASHING IN EYES

A. Immediate symptoms

1. Mechanical irritation
2. Watering of eyes
3. Inflammation of conjunctivas

B. First aid: see **blue** pages, section **6**

CALCIUM CHLORIDE
POTASSIUM CHLORIDE
SODIUM BICARBONATE
SODIUM CHLORIDE

These soluble salts are either nontoxic or have a very low level of toxicity.

Their concentrated aqueous solutions, however, may be slightly caustic (corrosive) and affect mucous membranes of the digestive system and eyes.

I. INHALATION

Only when large amounts of fine dust are inhaled will the following symptoms occur:

A. Symptoms of acute poisoning

1. Slight irritation of nose
2. Sneezing

B. First aid: see **yellow** pages, section **6**

II. INGESTION

A. Symptoms of acute poisoning

1. Disagreeable taste
2. Nausea and vomiting
3. Gastro-intestinal irritation (CALCIUM CHLORIDE only)

B. First aid: see **green** pages, section **8**

III. SKIN CONTACT

Only concentrated solutions that remain in contact with healthy skin for some time may cause

A. Immediate symptoms

1. Irritation
2. Inflammation
3. Small ulcerations

B. First aid: see **pink** pages, section **2**

IV. SPLASHING IN EYES

A. Immediate symptoms

1. Mechanical irritation
2. Watering of eyes
3. Inflammation of conjunctivas

B. First aid: see **blue** pages, section **6**

ALUMINUM (dust)
(Aluminum hydrate)
ALUMINUM HYDROXIDE
ALUMINUM OXIDE
ASBESTOS
CALCIUM CARBONATE
CARBON
CARBON BLACK
KAOLIN
POLY(VINYL CHLORIDE)
SILICA
TALC
TITANIUM (dust)
TITANIUM OXIDE
TUNGSTEN CARBIDE

These substances are solid, amorphous, and completely nontoxic to the organism that shows no immediate toxic symptoms. POLY(VINYL CHLORIDE) decomposes under heat, giving off hydrochloric acid fumes (see HYDROCHLORIC ACID, **white** pages, section **1**, page 31).

ASBESTOS and SILICA have been recognized in the United States as having serious injurious effects on the lungs in both long and short range, particularly the former. Criteria documents discussing both from many aspects are available from the Superintendent of Documents, U.S. Government Printing Office, Washington, D.C. 20402

OCCUPATIONAL EXPOSURE TO ASBESTOS – HSM – 72–10267, 2nd printing, 1972.
OCCUPATIONAL EXPOSURE TO CRYSTALLINE SILICA – HEW, Publication No. (NIOSH) 75–120, 1974.

I. INHALATION

A. Symptoms of heavy inhalation

1. Sneezing
2. Slight irritation of nose

B. First aid: see **yellow** pages, section **6**

II. INGESTION

No symptoms

First aid: see **green** pages, section **10**

III. SKIN CONTACT

No symptoms

First aid: see **pink** pages, section 7

IV. SPLASHING IN EYES

A. Immediate symptoms

1. Mechanical irritation
2. Watering of eyes
3. Inflammation of conjunctivas

B. First aid: see **blue** pages, section 7

(Alkylmercury compounds)
DIETHYLMERCURY
DIMETHYLMERCURY
ETHYLMERCURY
ETHYLMERCURIC CHLORIDE
ETHYLMERCURIC HYDROXIDE
MERCURY (organic compounds)
MERCURY FULMINATE
METHYLMERCURY
METHYLMERCURY BORATE
METHYLMERCURY HYDROXIDE
METHYLMERCURY IODIDE
METHYLMERCURY NITRATE
METHYLMERCURY PHOSPHATE
PHENYLMERCURIC ACETATE
PHENYLMERCURY
PHENYLMERCURY OLEATE

These substances are all toxic on inhalation, ingestion, or contact with skin. They cause lesions in the organs and particularly the nervous system.

They are toxic on acute or chronic exposure.

All cases of poisoning by these substances, even if they are not serious, must be reported to the physician, who alone is competent to treat the victim.

I. INHALATION

A. Symptoms of acute poisoning

1. Metallic taste
2. Salivation
3. Headache
4. Dizziness
5. Clumsiness, lack of coordination
6. General weakness
7. Trembling of arms and legs (occasionally)
8. Convulsions

B. First aid: see **yellow** pages, section **5**

II. INGESTION

In addition to the symptoms mentioned under I. INHALATION

A. Symptoms of acute poisoning

1. Irritation of mouth and throat
2. Stomach pains
3. Nausea and vomiting
4. Diarrhea

B. First aid: see **green** pages, section **9**

III. SKIN CONTACT

All organic derivatives of mercury are absorbed by healthy skin and may cause chronic poisoning.

A. Immediate symptoms

1. Irritation
2. Itching
3. Redness
4. Blisters
5. Ulcerations (MERCURY FULMINATE only)

B. First aid: see **pink** pages, section **2**

IV. SPLASHING IN EYES

A. Immediate symptoms

1. Irritation
2. Watering of eyes
3. Irritation of conjunctivas
4. Serious lesions may occur in eyes

B. First aid: see **blue** pages, section **6**

MERCURIC CHLORIDE
MERCURIC IODIDE
MERCUROUS CHLORIDE
MERCUROUS IODIDE
MERCURY (metal)
MERCURY (soluble salts)
MERCURY ACETATE
MERCURY NITRATE (acid)
MERCURY OXYCYANIDE

Except for metallic mercury, whose vapors are sufficiently volatile to cause very severe poisoning, the soluble mercury salts are all toxic to tissues and, in addition to their severe toxicity, cause hydrargyrism on exposure over long periods. Hydrargyrism has highly characteristic symptoms but is not discussed in this manual.

I. INHALATION

A. Symptoms of very acute poisoning (mercury vapors)

1. Metallic taste
2. Rapid and difficult breathing
3. Coughing
4. Bronchitis followed by chemical pneumonia (diagnosis can only be made by a physician)
5. Risk of acute pulmonary edema (for up to 15 days)

B. Symptoms of acute poisoning

After 2 days

1. Evil-smelling salivation
2. Inflammation of mouth
3. Profuse sweating
4. Headache
5. Nausea, vomiting

6. Stomach cramps
7. Diarrhea
8. Great weakness

C. First aid: see **yellow** pages, section **5**

II. INGESTION

A. Immediate symptoms

1. Metallic taste
2. Intense thirst
3. Pain in swallowing
4. Stomach or abdominal pain
5. Nausea and vomiting; vomit may contain blood or greenish substance
6. Diarrhea, occasionally blood-stained or greenish
7. State of shock
   - weak and rapid pulse
   - cold sweat—pale complexion
   - tendency to fainting
   - cold hands and feet
8. Trembling of arms and legs

B. First aid: see **green** pages, section **2**

III. SKIN CONTACT

The soluble mercury salts are irritating to the skin.
They may also penetrate healthy skin.*

*Metallic mercury is not irritating but may be absorbed through healthy skin.

A. Immediate symptoms

1. Irritation
2. Inflammation
3. Blisters

B. First aid: see **pink** pages, section **2**

IV. SPLASHING IN EYES

Metallic mercury is not irritating. Insoluble mercury salts are mechanical irritants while soluble salts are chemical irritants to the mucous membranes.

A. Immediate symptoms

1. Irritation
2. Watering of eyes
3. Inflammation of conjunctivas
4. Edema of eyelids
5. Occasionally serious lesions in eyes

B. First aid: see **blue** pages, section **6**

17

ALLYL ALCOHOL
ALLYL CHLORIDE
ALLYL GLYCIDYL ETHER
DIEPOXYBUTANE
DIGLYCIDYLETHER
EPICHLOROHYDRIN
ETHYL ACRYLATE
ETHYLENE OXIDE
GLYCIDOL
GLYCIDYL ACRYLATE
ISOCYANATES
METHYL ACRYLATE
NICKEL (fumes and dust)
NICKEL CARBONYL
PROPYLENE OXIDE
STYRENE

These substances are all irritating to the respiratory organs, skin, and mucous membranes of the digestive system and eyes. Some of them have a toxic effect on the liver and kidneys.

I. INHALATION

A. Symptoms of very acute poisoning

1. Irritation of mucous membranes (nose, eyes, throat)
2. Watering of eyes and coryza
3. Thoracic congestion
4. Difficulty in breathing
5. Coughing
6. BLUISH face and lips
7. Chemical bronchitis (diagnosis can only be made by a physician)
8. Risk of acute pulmonary edema

B. Symptoms of acute poisoning

1. Irritation of mucous membranes (nose, eyes)
2. Headache
3. Nausea, occasionally vomiting

4. BLUISH face and lips
5. Dizziness
6. Fatigue
7. Diarrhea

C. First aid: see **yellow** pages, section **4**

II. INGESTION

Because of their pungent smell, there is little risk of ingestion of these substances.

A. Symptoms of acute poisoning

1. Irritation of lips, mouth, and throat
2. Pain in swallowing
3. Stomach and abdominal pain
4. Nausea and vomiting
5. Diarrhea
6. State of shock
   - weak and rapid pulse
   - cold sweat—pale complexion
   - tendency to fainting
   - cold hands and feet
7. Convulsions may occur
8. Risk of acute pulmonary edema

B. First aid: see **green** pages, section **2**

III. CONTACT WITH MOIST SKIN

These substances all penetrate healthy skin and are highly irritating to moist skin.

A. Immediate symptoms

1. Itching and irritation (except with ETHYLENE OXIDE and PROPYLENE OXIDE)
2. Inflammation
3. Blisters that may be very large, although painless at first
4. Burns and painful ulcerations (NICKEL CARBONYL and ALLYL ALCOHOL only)

B. First aid: see **pink** pages, section **6**

IV. SPLASHING IN EYES

A. Immediate symptoms

1. Irritation
2. Watering of eyes
3. Inflammation of conjunctivas
4. Chemical burns in corneas
5. Possibility of serious lesions in eyes

B. First aid: see **blue** pages, section **5**

DIBUTYLLEAD
DIETHYLLEAD
LEAD OLEATE
LEAD PHENATE
LEAD PHTHALATE
LEAD STEARATE
TETRAETHYLLEAD*†
TETRAMETHYLLEAD*†
TRIBUTYLLEAD*†
TRIETHYLLEAD*†
TRIMETHYLLEAD*†

*volatile substances
†probably dimers

These organic lead compounds can all be absorbed by healthy skin. In cases of severe exposure, they are toxic to the nervous system, liver, and kidneys.

In the case of inhalation, ingestion, and skin contact over prolonged periods, they cause chronic lead poisoning (saturnism).

They are highly caustic (corrosive), volatile liquids or gases.

I. INHALATION

The risk of severe poisoning depends on the volatility of the compounds (see substances with *).

A. Symptoms of acute poisoning

1. Occasional irritation of nose
2. Shivering
3. Restlessness
4. Delirium
5. Convulsions

B. Symptoms of mild poisoning

1. Restlessness
2. Trembling of hands
3. Headache

4. Pale complexion
5. Occasionally nausea and vomiting
6. Insomnia and nightmares

C. First aid: see **yellow** pages, section **5**

II. INGESTION

A. Symptoms of acute poisoning

See I. INHALATION

B. First aid: see **green** pages, section **9**

III. SKIN CONTACT

A. Immediate symptoms

1. Itching
2. Inflammation
3. Blisters

B. First aid: see **pink** pages, section **6**

IV. SPLASHING IN EYES

A. Immediate symptoms

1. Irritation
2. Watering of eyes
3. Inflammation of conjunctivas

B. First aid: see **blue** pages, section **6**

ALIPHATIC AMINES
AMMONIA
AMMONIUM HYDROXIDE
(Ammonia water)
BUTYLAMINES
DIBUTYLAMINES
DIETHYLAMINE
DIMETHYLAMINE
DIPROPYLAMINES
ETHYLAMINE
METHYLAMINE
PROPYLAMINES
TRIETHYLAMINE
TRIMETHYLAMINE

Aqueous solutions of these substances are highly irritating to mucous membranes of the respiratory and digestive systems, eyes, and to healthy skin.

I. INHALATION

A. Symptoms of very acute poisoning

1. Irritation of nose, throat, and eyes
2. Burning sensation
3. Difficulty in breathing
4. Fits of coughing
5. Chemical pneumonia or bronchitis
6. Acute pulmonary edema

(5–6: diagnosis can only be made by a physician)

7. Sudden death (AMMONIA only)

B. Symptoms of acute poisoning

1. Irritation of nose and eyes
2. Sneezing
3. Tingling sensation in respiratory tract
4. Coughing
5. Risk of chemical bronchitis

AFTER AN APPARENT ARREST IN THE SYMPTOMS

6. Risk of acute pulmonary edema

C. First aid: see **yellow** pages, section **1**

II. INGESTION

A. Symptoms of acute poisoning

1. Immediate burning sensation in mouth, throat, and stomach (the buccal [cheeks and mouth cavity] mucous membranes are attacked)
2. Pain in swallowing
3. Edema of the glottis (diagnosis can only be made by a physician)
4. Strong salivation
5. Nausea and vomiting of blood
6. Stomach cramps
7. Rapid breathing
8. State of shock
   - weak and rapid pulse
   - cold sweat—pale complexion
   - tendency to fainting
   - cold hands and feet
9. Diarrhea, occasionally blood-stained
10. Risk of stomach perforation

B. First aid: see **green** pages, section 3

III. SKIN CONTACT

A. Immediate symptoms

1. Itching and tingling sensation
2. Painful burning
3. Painful ulcerations

4. State of shock
   - weak and rapid pulse
   - cold sweat—pale complexion
   - tendency to fainting
   - cold hands and feet

B. First aid: see **pink** pages, section **4**

IV. SPLASHING IN EYES

A. Immediate symptoms

1. Immediate, highly painful irritation of eyes and eyelids
2. Intense watering of eyes
3. Victim keeps eyelids tightly closed
4. Burns and irreparable damage to mucous membranes of eyes
5. Serious lesions in eyes

B. First aid: see **blue** pages, section **2**

AMMONIUM CARBONATE
CALCIUM HYDROXIDE
LITHIUM CARBONATE
MILK OF LIME
POTASSIUM CARBONATE
SODIUM CARBONATE
SODIUM SILICATE
TRISODIUM PHOSPHATE (Na_3PO_4)

In contact with water, the above crystalline substances give alkaline solutions that are highly irritating to mucous membranes of the respiratory and digestive systems and eyes.

LITHIUM CARBONATE is toxic to the kidneys.

I. INHALATION

A. Symptoms of very acute poisoning

1. Irritation of nose, eyes, and throat
2. Sneezing
3. Difficulty in breathing
4. Coughing, occasional fits of coughing
5. Chemical bronchitis (diagnosis can only be made by a physician)

B. Symptoms of acute poisoning

1. Irritation of nose and eyes
2. Tingling sensation in respiratory tract
3. Sneezing
4. Coughing

C. First aid: see **yellow** pages, section **2**

II. INGESTION

A. Symptoms of acute poisoning

1. Burning sensation in mouth, esophagus, and stomach

2. Irritation of mouth
3. Pain in swallowing
4. Stomach cramps
5. Nausea and vomiting (LITHIUM CARBONATE only)
6. Occasional trembling of arms and legs (LITHIUM CARBONATE only)
7. Occasional mental confusion (LITHIUM CARBONATE only)

B. First aid: see **green** pages, section **3**

III. CONTACT WITH MOIST SKIN

A. Immediate symptoms

1. Itching and tingling sensation
2. Burning sensation
3. Inflammation

B. First aid: see **pink** pages, section **9**

IV. SPLASHING IN EYES

A. Immediate symptoms

1. Mechanical irritation, followed by chemical irritation
2. Pain
3. Watering of eyes
4. Risk of serious lesions in eyes if victim keeps eyelids tightly closed

B. First aid: see **blue** pages, section **3**

ARSENIC (soluble salts)
ARSENIC TRICHLORIDE
ARSINE (gas)
PHOSPHINE
PHOSPHORUS CHLORIDES
PHOSPHORUS PENTACHLORIDE
PHOSPHORUS TRICHLORIDE

ARSINE and PHOSPHINE are highly toxic gases.

The liquid chlorides give off highly irritating and toxic fumes.

All the above are toxic to the blood, liver, and kidneys and may cause sequelae of these organs.

I. INHALATION

A. Symptoms of very acute poisoning

1. Passing attack of headache
2. Sudden loss of consciousness
3. Almost instantaneous death

B. Symptoms of acute poisoning

1. Headache
2. Dizziness
3. Nausea, occasionally vomiting
4. Fatigue
5. Difficulty in breathing
6. Pale or bluish face
7. Dry cough
8. Cold sweat
9. Abdominal pain with diarrhea
10. Trembling of arms and legs
11. Convulsions
12. Loss of consciousness
13. Risk of pulmonary edema
14. Death

C. First aid: see **yellow** pages, section **1**

II. INGESTION

A. Symptoms of acute poisoning

In addition to the severe symptoms given under I. INHALATION, B

1. Irritation of mouth and throat
2. Burning pains in stomach
3. Nausea and vomiting
4. Burning and fetid diarrhea

B. First aid: see **green** pages, section **1**

III. SKIN CONTACT

These compounds all penetrate or react with healthy skin and cause general poisoning even when there is limited contact with the skin. In addition, the chlorides are highly irritating to tissues.

In addition to the general symptoms described under I. INHALATION.

A. Immediate symptoms

1. Painful irritation
2. Inflammation
3. Blisters
4. Rapid ulceration of the skin

B. First aid: see **pink** pages, section **1**
see **pink** pages, section **2** (ARSENIC [soluble salts] only)

IV. SPLASHING IN EYES

A. Immediate symptoms

1. Immediate irritation of eyes
2. Watering of eyes
3. Inflammation and burning sensation
4. Risk of serious lesions in eyes

B. First aid: see **blue** pages, section **1**
see **blue** pages, section **6** (ARSENIC [soluble salts] only)

(Alkyltin compounds)
DIBUTYLTIN
DIETHYLTIN
DIHEXYLTIN
DIIODODIETHYLTIN
DIMETHYLTIN
DIOCTYLTIN
TETRABUTYLTIN
TETRAETHYLTIN
TETRAISOALKYLTINS
TETRAPENTYLTIN
TETRAPROPYLTIN
TIN (organic compounds)
TRIBUTYLTIN*
TRIETHYLTIN*
TRIMETHYLTIN*
TRIPHENYLTIN*
TRIPROPYLTIN*

*probably dimers

The above substances are all toxic to the nervous system and cause sequelae, in addition to lesions in the liver and kidneys. Their toxicity increases with decreasing molecular weight.

I. INHALATION

A. Symptoms of very acute poisoning

1. Irritation of nose and eyes
2. Sneezing
3. Headache
4. Nausea
5. General feeling of discomfort
6. Coughing

B. First aid: see **yellow** pages, section **5**

II. INGESTION

A. Symptoms of acute poisoning

1. Irritation of digestive system
2. Headache
3. Nausea and vomiting
4. Stomach pains
5. Dizziness

6. Convulsions
7. Loss of consciousness
8. Coma
9. Death or risk of permanent paralysis

B. First aid: see **green** pages, section **9**

III. SKIN CONTACT

These substances are irritating to the skin in varying degrees.

A. Immediate symptoms

1. Itching
2. Irritation
3. Inflammation
4. Blisters may occur, followed by ulceration of the skin

B. First aid: see **pink** pages, section **2**

IV. SPLASHING IN EYES

Vapors of these substances are irritating to the eyes.

A. Immediate symptoms

1. Irritation
2. Watering of eyes
3. Inflammation of conjunctivas

B. First aid: see **blue** pages, section **6**

23

CHLORTHION
DDVP
DEMETON
DIAZINON
DIPTEREX
EPN
ISOPESTOX
MALATHION
METHYL PARATHION
OMPA
ORGANOPHOSPHORUS COMPOUNDS
PARAOXON
PARATHION
PHOSDRIN
PHOSPHORIC ESTERS
RONNEL
SULFOTEPP
TEPP
TRITHION

The ORGANOPHOSPHORUS COMPOUNDS are volatile, extremely toxic compounds with **very rapid effects**.

They block the cholinesterase of the blood, which results in nervous disorders (hypervagotonia) and serious muscular disturbances, as well as increased secretions (saliva, sweat).

NOTE: A splash of a single drop of PARATHION in the eye may result in serious disorders, and even death.

I. INHALATION

A. Symptoms of acute poisoning

1st phase (muscarinic)

1. Profuse salivation
2. Nausea and vomiting
3. Stomach cramps
4. Diarrhea
5. Headache and dizziness
6. Troubled breathing (asthmatic)
7. Very small pupils (myosis)
8. Anxiety and agitation

2nd phase (nicotinic)

a. Muscular disorders

1. Muscle contractions that first occur in the face and subsequently spread throughout the body
2. Convulsions
3. Decreasing muscle power

b. Respiratory disorders

1. Heavy cough
2. Hypersecretion of the bronchia
3. Weakness of respiratory muscles

c. Disorders of the heart

1. Weak and slow pulse
2. Irregular pulse

3rd phase (terminal)

1. High fever
2. Loss of consciousness
3. Death

B. First aid: see **yellow** pages, section **3**

II. INGESTION

A. Symptoms of acute poisoning

See symptoms described under I. INHALATION

B. First aid: see **green** pages, section **5**

III. SKIN CONTACT

The ORGANOPHOSPHORUS COMPOUNDS are capable of rapidly penetrating healthy skin.

A. Immediate symptoms

See symptoms described under I. INHALATION

B. First aid: see **pink** pages, section **11**

IV. SPLASHING IN EYES

The ORGANOPHOSPHORUS COMPOUNDS are rapidly absorbed by mucous membranes of the eyes and cause general poisoning within a short period of time.

A. Immediate symptoms

1. Irritation
2. Watering of eyes

These are quickly followed by the symptoms described under I. INHALATION

B. First aid: see **blue** pages, section **9**

LEAD (metal fumes)
LEAD ACETATE
LEAD ANTIMONATE
LEAD ARSENATE
LEAD CARBONATE
LEAD CHLORIDE
LEAD CHROMATE (red)
LEAD CHROMATE (yellow)
LEAD DIOXIDE
LEAD NITRATE
LEAD OXIDE (PbO)
LEAD OXIDE (red)
LEAD OXYCHLORIDE
LEAD SUBACETATE
LEAD SULFIDE

Only LEAD SULFATE is acknowledged to be **nontoxic**. The other substances are toxic to the kidneys, nerves, muscles, and blood. The water-soluble salts and the oxides react with gastric juices (HCl) and cause gastro-intestinal irritation and lead poisoning.

As a result of inhalation, ingestion, and skin contact, these substances may eventually cause chronic lead poisoning (saturnism).

I. INHALATION

Poisoning may be caused by these compounds in the form of fine dust as well as by their decomposition products obtained during heating or cleaning.

A. Symptoms of acute poisoning

1. Slight irritation of nose and eyes
2. Headache
3. Stomach cramps
4. Fatigue

B. First aid: see **yellow** pages, section **6**

II. INGESTION

A. Symptoms of acute poisoning

1. Metallic taste in mouth

2. Constriction of throat
3. Stomach pains
4. Nausea and vomiting, occasionally of blood
5. Spasmodic abdominal pain
6. Diarrhea
7. Convulsions
8. Coma
9. Death

B. First aid: see **green** pages, section **2**

III. SKIN CONTACT

A. Immediate symptoms

1. Irritation
2. Inflammation

B. First aid: see **pink** pages, section **2**

IV. SPLASHING IN EYES

The insoluble salts of lead are mechanical irritants whereas the soluble salts are chemical irritants to the eyes.

A. Immediate symptoms

1. Mechanical or chemical irritation
2. Watering of eyes
3. Inflammation of conjunctivas

B. First aid: see **blue** pages, section **6**

25

ACETONE CYANOHYDRIN
ACRYLONITRILE
BITTER ALMOND ESSENCE
CHERRY LAUREL WATER
CYANOGEN CHLORIDE
FERRICYANIDES (K, Na)
FERROCYANIDES (K, Na)
HYDROCYANIC ACID
NITROFERRICYANIDES
POTASSIUM CYANIDE
SODIUM CYANIDE

HYDROCYANIC ACID, POTASSIUM CYANIDE, and SODIUM CYANIDE are highly toxic substances that interfere with the respiration of the living cells. This can be the result of either inhalation or ingestion.

ACRYLONITRILE is toxic when inhaled and highly irritating to skin and eyes.

The FERRICYANIDES and FERROCYANIDES are less toxic.

I. INHALATION

A. Symptoms of very acute poisoning (HYDROCYANIC ACID only)

1. Victim cries out before losing consciousness
2. Victim falls to the ground
3. Wheezing
4. Foaming at mouth
5. Violent convulsions
6. Almost immediate death

B. Symptoms of acute poisoning

1. Excitement phase

— headache

— breath smells of bitter almond

— dizziness

— nausea, occasionally vomiting

— rapid breathing

2. Depression phase

— difficulty in breathing

— pain in area around heart

— anguish

3. Convulsion phase

— convulsions

— jaws clenched together

— foaming at mouth

— loss of consciousness

4. Paralysis phase

— prolonged coma

— dilated pupils

— weak and irregular pulse

— breathing stops

— death

If the subject survives, there is risk of nervous sequelae.

C. Symptoms of slight poisoning

1. Headache
2. Dizziness
3. Anguish

4. Difficulty in breathing

D. First aid: see **yellow** pages, section **8**

II. INGESTION

See symptoms described under I. INHALATION, B and C.

First aid: see **green** pages, section **11**

III. SKIN CONTACT

The gaseous and liquid compounds are quickly absorbed by the skin and cause symptoms described under I. INHALATION, B and C.

Depending on their nature, they can be very or only slightly irritating.

First aid: see **pink** pages, section **8**

IV. SPLASHING IN EYES

When absorbed by mucous membranes of the eyes, these compounds can cause the same symptoms described in I. INHALATION, C.

A. Immediate symptoms

1. Irritation
2. Watering of eyes

B. First aid: see **blue** pages, section **5**

DINITROCRESOLS
DINITROPHENOLS
DNBP
DNOC
ETHYLENE GLYCOL DINITRATE
ETHYL NITRATE
METHYL NITRATE
NITROGLYCERIN
NITROPHENOLS
PENTACHLOROPHENATES
PENTACHLOROPHENOL
PROPYL NITRATE

These nitro-organic or chlorophenolic compounds may inhibit phosphate bonds and consequently interfere with cellular respiration, which causes high fever.

They are irritating to lungs, skin, and eyes and may cause lesions in liver and kidneys.

I. INHALATION

A. Symptoms of acute poisoning

1. Irritation of nose
2. Nausea and vomiting
3. Coughing
4. High fever
5. Profuse sweating
6. Rapid, difficult breathing
7. BLUISH face and lips; YELLOW in the case of DINITROCRESOLS only
8. Intense fatigue
9. Dizziness
10. Convulsions
11. Loss of consciousness
12. Death due to heart failure
13. Risk of severe pulmonary edema if victim survives

B. First aid: see **yellow** pages, section **4**

II. INGESTION

A. Symptoms of acute poisoning

1. Burning sensation in mouth and throat
2. Salivation
3. Dizziness
4. Nausea and vomiting
5. High fever
6. Profuse sweating
7. Rapid and difficult breathing
8. BLUISH face and lips; YELLOW in the case of DNOC only
9. Intense fatigue
10. Convulsions
11. Lack of consciousness
12. Death
13. Risk of pulmonary edema if victim survives

B. First aid: see **green** pages, section 7

III. SKIN CONTACT

These substances can all be absorbed through healthy skin, especially when they are dissolved in organic solvents. They may cause delayed symptoms identical to those described under I. INHALATION.

A. Immediate symptoms

1. Irritation

2. Inflammation
3. Blisters

B. Delayed symptoms

See I. INHALATION

C. First aid: see **pink** pages, section **6**

IV. SPLASHING IN EYES

A. Immediate symptoms

1. Burning pain in eyes
2. Irritation
3. Watering of eyes
4. Inflammation of conjunctivas

B. First aid: see **blue** pages, section **3**

DISODIUM PHOSPHATE
MAGNESIUM CHLORIDE
MAGNESIUM SULFATE
SODIUM SULFATE
SODIUM THIOCYANATE
SODIUM THIOSULFATE

These compounds are crystalline, water-soluble, and considered nontoxic and nonirritating to skin and mucous membranes.

Except for SODIUM THIOCYANATE they are laxatives and consequently used as first aid to accelerate the elimination of toxic products from the intestines. MAGNESIUM SULFATE and SODIUM SULFATE are most frequently used.

I. INHALATION

First aid: see **yellow** pages, section **6**

II. INGESTION

No risk

III. SKIN CONTACT

Although these substances are not irritating to skin, it is advisable to avoid prolonged contact of the skin with them in powder form or concentrated solutions.

First aid: see **pink** pages, section **7**
see **pink** pages, section **8** (THIOCYANATES only)

IV. SPLASHING IN EYES

A. Immediate symptoms

1. Mechanical irritation

2. Watering of eyes

B. First aid: see **blue** pages, section **6**
see **blue** pages, section **5** (THIOCYANATES only)

(Alkylaluminum compounds)
ALUMINUM ALKYLS
DIETHYLALUMINUM CHLORIDE
DIETHYLALUMINUM HYDRIDE
TRIETHYLALUMINUM
TRIISOBUTYLALUMINUM
TRIMETHYLALUMINUM

These substances occur as liquids at normal temperatures. They are generally diluted with a hydrocarbon-type solvent and kept in a nitrogen atmosphere according to very strict safety regulations.

These compounds burst spontaneously and almost instantaneously into flames as soon as they come into contact with atmospheric oxygen or water and give off nontoxic fumes of ALUMINUM OXIDE (see **white** pages, section **14,** page 73).

I. INHALATION OF FUMES

A. Symptoms of acute inhalation

1. Sneezing
2. Slight irritation of nose

B. First aid: see **yellow** pages, section **6**

II. INGESTION

No risk because of strict handling requirements.

III. SKIN CONTACT

Little risk because of the protective equipment required during handling of the product.

Ignition of the product.

A. Immediate symptoms

1. Third-degree burns (irreparable damage to tissues)
2. State of shock
   - weak and rapid pulse
   - cold sweat—pale complexion
   - tendency to fainting
   - cold hands and feet
3. Loss of consciousness
4. Death

B. First aid: see **pink** pages, section **10**

IV. SPLASHING IN EYES

Little risk because of the protective equipment required during handling of the product.

A. Immediate symptoms

1. Burning, by flames, of face and eyelids
2. Excruciating pain
3. Swelling of eyelids
4. Possible injury of eyes and impairment of vision

B. First aid: see **blue** pages, section **8**

ALKANES (solids)
CHLORONAPHTHALENES
DIPHENYL
DIPHENYLAMINE
NAPHTHALENE
NAPHTHYLAMINES
PARAFFINS (solid compounds)
PHENYLNAPHTHYLAMINES

These substances are solid or have a waxy appearance and are soluble in organic solvents. They are considered to present no risk on severe exposure.

alpha-Naphthylamine and *beta*-Naphthylamine are listed by the Occupational Safety and Health Administration as "cancer-suspect agents." See GENERAL INDUSTRY, OSHA SAFETY AND HEALTH STANDARDS, 29 CFR 1910.

I. INHALATION OF DUST

A. Symptoms of severe poisoning

1. Irritation of nose
2. Headache
3. Nausea may occur
4. Coughing

B. First aid: see **yellow** pages, section **2**

II. INGESTION

Only the amines in the list above are slightly irritating to mucous membranes of the digestive system.

A. Symptoms of severe poisoning

1. Slight irritation of stomach

2. Nausea, occasionally vomiting
3. Diarrhea
4. General fatigue

B. First aid: see **green** pages, section **10**

III. SKIN CONTACT

In solution in organic solvents, these substances will slowly penetrate the skin. The immediate symptoms that can be observed are the result of poisoning by the solvent used.

First aid: see **pink** pages, section **9**

IV. SPLASHING IN EYES

A. Immediate symptoms

1. Mechanical irritation
2. Watering of eyes

B. First aid: see **blue** pages, section **6**

DIPYRIDYL CHLORIDE
DIPYRIDYL DIMETHYL SULFATE
DIQUAT
(Gramoxon)
PARAQUAT
QUARTERNARY AMMONIUM COMPOUNDS

The pesticides belonging to the dipyridyl group are not volatile. Their solutions are highly toxic when inhaled, and particularly when ingested, while resorption through healthy skin is relatively slow.

They are irritating to eyes, and toxic to liver, kidneys, and lungs.

I. INHALATION

A. Symptoms of acute poisoning

1. Irritation of nose and eyes
2. Sneezing
3. Nose bleed
4. Painful obstruction of throat

B. First aid: see **yellow** pages, section **4**

II. INGESTION

A. Symptoms of acute poisoning

1. Burning sensation in mouth and throat
2. Irritation of mucous membranes
3. Difficulty in swallowing
4. Burning sensation in stomach
5. Nausea and vomiting, possibly of blood

6. Painful abdominal cramps
7. Diarrhea, may be blood-stained
8. There is risk of serious lesions in
   - the liver
   - the kidneys
   - the lungs (fatal chemical pneumonia)

B. First aid: see **green** pages, section **5**

III. SKIN CONTACT

A. Immediate symptoms

1. Irritation
2. Inflammation
3. Painful blisters

B. First aid: see **pink** pages, section **6**

IV. SPLASHING IN EYES

A. Immediate symptoms

1. Painful burning sensation
2. Watering of eyes
3. Inflammation
4. Sensitiveness to bright light

B. First aid: see **blue** pages, section **5**

First aid **IN CASE OF INHALATION OF**

ACETALDEHYDE
ACETIC ACID
ACETIC ANHYDRIDE
ACROLEIN
ALIPHATIC AMINES
AMMONIA
AMMONIUM HYDROXIDE
(Ammonia water)
ARSENIC (soluble salts)
ARSENIC TRICHLORIDE
ARSINE (gas)
BROMINE
BUTYLAMINES
BUTYRALDEHYDE
CHLORINE
CHLORINE DIOXIDE
CHLOROACETIC ACID
DIBUTYLAMINES
DIETHYLAMINE
DIMETHYLAMINE
DIPROPYLAMINES
ETHYLAMINE
ETHYL CHLOROFORMATE
FLUORINE
FLUOSILICIC ACID
FORMALDEHYDE
FORMIC ACID
HYDRIODIC ACID
HYDROBROMIC ACID
HYDROCHLORIC ACID
HYDROFLUORIC ACID
(Hydrogen chloride)
HYDROGEN PEROXIDE
HYDROGEN SELENIDE
HYDROGEN SULFIDE
IODINE
ISOBUTYRALDEHYDE
METHYLAMINE
METHYL CHLOROFORMATE
NITRIC ACID
OSMIC ACID
OZONE
PERACETIC ACID
PERCHLORIC ACID
PHENOL
PHOSGENE
PHOSPHINE
PHOSPHORIC ACID
PHOSPHORUS CHLORIDES
PHOSPHORUS PENTACHLORIDE
PHOSPHORUS TRICHLORIDE
POTASSIUM CHLORITE
POTASSIUM FLUORIDE
PROPIONALDEHYDE
PROPYLAMINES
SODIUM CHLORITE
SODIUM FLUORIDE
SULFUR DIOXIDE
SULFURIC ACID
SULFUROUS ACID
SULFUR TRIOXIDE
TRICHLOROACETIC ACID
TRIETHYLAMINE
TRIMETHYLAMINE

— First aiders must take precautions for their own safety if they must enter the contaminated area to help the victim.

— Always remove the victim from the contaminated area.

— Notify a physician immediately and inform him of
  - the nature of the substance inhaled and
  - the state of the victim and, if possible, his symptoms.

— Prevent the victim from making any unnecessary exertion or movement.
— Never give an unconscious person anything to drink.

A. If the victim is conscious,

1. Remove him from the contaminated area to a quiet, cool, and well-ventilated area.
2. Lay him down with his legs raised.
3. Loosen his collar and belt.
4. Cover him with a blanket.
5. Calm and reassure him.

B. If the victim coughs a great deal,

(in addition to the measures recommended in A)

6. Make him inhale from a gauze pad soaked with
   - a little ethyl alcohol or
   - a few drops of ether.

   } CAUTION! These liquids are flammable.
7. Make him inhale oxygen under low pressure with a PULMOTOR or similar type of equipment.*

C. If the victim is unconscious but breathing,

(in addition to the measures recommended in A)

8. Remove dentures or partial plates.
9. Make him inhale oxygen under low pressure with a PULMOTOR or similar type of equipment* until physician arrives.

D. If the victim has stopped breathing,

1. Remove him as quickly as possible from the contaminated area.

*See Vital Equipment, page 4.

2. Quickly
   - lay him down on his stomach on a blanket
   - loosen his collar and belt
   - begin artificial respiration (Holger-Nielsen method); be very gentle to avoid injuring his lungs.
3. As soon as possible, administer oxygen under low pressure with a PULMOTOR or similar type of equipment.*
4. Continue this treatment until the physician arrives or the victim begins to breathe unaided.
5. As soon as the victim begins to breathe or to move lay him down with his body raised and continue to administer oxygen.

NOTE: The physician will keep the victim under medical supervision for at least 2 days as there is risk of acute pulmonary edema or microbial infection.

*See Vital Equipment, page 4.

IN CASE OF INHALATION OF

ALKANES (solids)
AMMONIUM CARBONATE
AMMONIUM CHLORATE
AMMONIUM PERCHLORATE
BARIUM (soluble salts)
BARIUM ACETATE
BARIUM CARBONATE
BARIUM CHLORIDE
BARIUM FLUORIDE
BARIUM HYDROXIDE
BARIUM NITRATE
BARIUM OXIDE
BARIUM SULFIDE
CALCIUM HYDROXIDE
CHLORONAPHTHALENES
DIPHENYL
DIPHENYLAMINE
LITHIUM CARBONATE
NAPHTHALENE
NAPHTHYLAMINES
OXALIC ACID
PARAFFINS (solid compounds)
PHENYLNAPHTHYLAMINES
POTASSIUM CARBONATE
POTASSIUM CHLORATE
POTASSIUM PERCHLORATE
SODIUM CARBONATE
SODIUM CHLORATE
SODIUM PERCHLORATE
SODIUM SILICATE
TRISODIUM PHOSPHATE

— Always remove the victim from the contaminated area.

— Refer victim to the medical center in all cases. Call a physician or the medical center in severe cases when the victim cannot be moved.

A. If the victim feels only irritation of the nose,

1. Make him blow his nose to remove the substance but discourage him from sniffling.
2. Send him to the dispensary or medical center.

B. If the victim is coughing badly,

1. Loosen his collar.
2. Make him inhale from a gauze pad soaked with
   - a little ethyl alcohol or
   - a few drops of ether.

   } CAUTION! These liquids are flammable.

IN CASE OF INHALATION OF

ACETONE
ACETYLENE (pure material)
ALIPHATIC ALCOHOLS
ALKANES (gases) (C_1 to C_4)
AMYL ACETATE
BENZENE
BUTADIENE
BUTANE
BUTANOL
BUTYL ACETATE
CARBON DIOXIDE
CARBON DIOXIDE SNOW
CARBON MONOXIDE
CARBON TETRACHLORIDE
CHLOROBENZENE
CHLORODIFLUOROETHANE
CHLORODIFLUOROMETHANE
CHLOROETHANES (Di-, Mono-)
CHLOROETHANES (Tri-, Tetra-)
CHLOROFLUOROETHANES
CHLOROFLUOROMETHANES
CHLOROFORM
CHLOROMETHANES (Mono-, Di-, Tri-, Tetra-)
CHLOROPENTAFLUORO-ETHANE
CHLOROPROPANES
CHLOROPROPENES
CHLOROTRIFLUORO-ETHYLENE
CHLOROTRIFLUORO-METHANE
CHLORTHION
CYCLOHEXANE
DDVP
DECANE
DECANOL
DEMETON
DIAZINON
DICHLOROBENZENES
DICHLORODIFLUORO-METHANE
DICHLOROETHANES
DICHLOROETHYLENES
DICHLOROFLUORO-METHANE
DICHLOROPROPANES
DICHLOROTETRAFLUORO-ETHANES
DIETHYLENE GLYCOL
DIFLUOROETHANES
DIFLUOROETHYLENES
DIFLUOROMETHANE
DIISOBUTYLCARBINOL
DIPTEREX
EPN
ETHANE
ETHYL ACETATE
ETHYL ALCOHOL
ETHYLENE
ETHYLENE GLYCOL
ETHYL ETHER
ETHYL FLUORIDE
ETHYLHEXYL ACETATE
FLUOROMETHANE
FREON 11, 12, 13, 14, 21, 22, 112, 113, 114, 115, 116, 142b, 143, 151a, 152a
GASOLINE
GLYCERIN
HEPTANE
HEPTANOL
HEXACHLOROETHANE
HEXAFLUOROETHANE
HEXANE
HEXANOL
ISOBUTYL ACETATE
ISOPESTOX
ISOPROPYL ACETATE
MALATHION
METHANE
METHYL ACETATE
METHYL ALCOHOL
METHYL CHLORIDE
(Methylchloroform)

METHYLENE CHLORIDE
METHYLENE FLUORIDE
METHYL PARATHION
NITROGEN
NONANE
OCTANE
OMPA
ORGANOPHOSPHORUS COMPOUNDS
PARAOXON
PARATHION
PENTACHLOROETHANE
PENTANE
PENTANOL
PETROLEUM ETHERS
PHOSDRIN
PHOSPHORIC ESTERS
PROPANE
PROPYL ACETATE
PROPYL ALCOHOLS
PROPYLENE
PROPYLENE GLYCOL
RONNEL
SULFOTEPP
TEPP
TETRACHLORODIFLUORO-ETHANES
TETRACHLOROETHANES
TETRACHLOROETHYLENE
TETRAFLUOROETHYLENE
TETRAFLUOROMETHANE
TOLUENE
TRICHLOROETHANES
TRICHLOROETHYLENE
TRICHLOROFLUORO-METHANE
TRICHLOROTRIFLUORO-ETHANES
TRIETHYLENE GLYCOL
TRIFLUOROETHANES
TRIFLUOROMETHANE
TRITHION
VINYL ACETATE
VINYL CHLORIDE
VINYL FLUORIDE
VINYLIDENE CHLORIDE
VINYLIDENE FLUORIDE
WHITE SPIRIT
XYLENES

— Never give an unconscious person anything to drink.

— Always remove the victim from the contaminated area.

A. If the victim is conscious,

1. Remove him from the contaminated area to a quiet, cool, and well-ventilated area.
2. Lay him down with his legs raised, if his **face is RED**. Lay him down flat on his back with his head turned to one side and his legs raised, if his **face is PALE**.
3. Loosen his collar and belt.
4. Cover him with a blanket.
5. Speak reassuringly to him.

6. Notify a physician and inform him of the nature of the substance inhaled.

B. If the victim is—conscious but has difficulty breathing,
—unconscious but breathing,

1. Notify a physician and inform him of the nature of the substance inhaled and the state of the victim.
2. Lay him down with his legs slightly raised.
3. Remove dentures or partial plates.
4. Loosen his collar and belt.
5. Cover him with a blanket.
6. Make him inhale oxygen under low pressure with a PULMOTOR or similar type of equipment* until the physician arrives.

C. If the victim is no longer breathing,

1. Act quickly, as described in B, but begin artificial respiration or mouth-to-mouth resuscitation **AS QUICKLY AS POSSIBLE.**
2. As soon as possible administer oxygen under low pressure with a PULMOTOR or similar type of equipment.*
3. Continue this treatment until the physician arrives.

NOTE: METHYL ALCOHOL: Medical supervision and a check of the victim's visual acuity is indispensable.

Chlorinated solvents: **It is expressly contra-indicated** to administer adrenalin to a victim of chlorinated solvent poisoning.

ORGANOPHOSPHORUS COMPOUNDS: A physician should be called immediately to treat the victim.

The physician will keep the victim under medical supervision for at least 2 days as there is risk of acute pulmonary edema.

*See Vital Equipment, page 4.

IN CASE OF INHALATION OF

ALLYL ALCOHOL
ALLYL CHLORIDE
ALLYL GLYCIDYL ETHER
ANILINE
CHLORONITROBENZENES
DIEPOXYBUTANE
DIGYLCIDYL ETHER
DIMETHYLANILINE
DINITROBENZENES
DINITROCRESOLS
DINITROPHENOLS
DIPYRIDYL CHLORIDE
DIPYRIDYL DIMETHYL SULFATE
DIQUAT
DNBP
DNOC
EPICHLOROHYDRIN
ETHYL ACRYLATE
ETHYLENE GLYCOL DINITRATE
ETHYLENE OXIDE
ETHYL NITRATE
GLYCIDOL
GLYCIDYL ACRYLATE
(Gramoxon)
ISOCYANATES
METHYL ACRYLATE
METHYL NITRATE
NICKEL (fumes and dust)
NICKEL CARBONYL
NITROANILINES
NITROBENZENE
NITROGLYCERIN
NITROPHENOLS
PARAQUAT
PENTACHLOROPHENATES
PENTACHLOROPHENOL
PHENYLHYDRAZINE
PHENYLHYDROXYLAMINE
PROPYLENE OXIDE
PROPYL NITRATE
QUATERNARY AMMONIUM COMPOUNDS
STYRENE
TOLUIDINES
TRINITROBENZENE
XYLIDINES

— Notify a physician immediately and inform him of
- the nature of the substance inhaled and
- the state of the victim and, if possible, his symptoms.

— Never give an unconscious person anything to drink.

— Always remove the victim from the contaminated area.

A. If the victim is conscious but his face is blue,

1. Remove him from the contaminated area to a quiet, cool, and well-ventilated area.
2. Lay him **flat on his back** with his head turned to one side and his legs raised.

3. Loosen his collar and belt.
4. Cover him with a blanket.
5. Administer oxygen under low pressure, using a PULMOTOR or similar type of equipment.* **Never make the victim inhale Carbogen** (mixture of oxygen and carbon dioxide).

B. If the victim is unconscious but breathing,

(in addition to the treatment recommended in A)

6. Remove dentures or partial plates.
7. Continue to administer oxygen until the physician arrives.

NOTE: The physician will keep the victim under medical supervision for 1 or 2 days.

*See Vital Equipment, page 4.

IN CASE OF INHALATION OF

(Alkylmercury compounds)
(Alkyltin compounds)
DIBUTYLLEAD
DIBUTYLTIN
DIETHYLLEAD
DIETHLMERCURY
DIETHYLTIN
DIHEXYLTIN
DIIODODIETHYLTIN
DIMETHYLMERCURY
DIMETHYLTIN
DIOCTYLTIN
ETHYLMERCURY
ETHYLMERCURIC CHLORIDE
ETHYLMERCURIC HYDROXIDE
LEAD OLEATE
LEAD PHENATE
LEAD PHTHALATE
LEAD STEARATE
MERCURIC CHLORIDE
MERCURIC IODIDE
MERCUROUS CHLORIDE
MERCUROUS IODIDE
MERCURY (metal)
MERCURY (organic compounds)
MERCURY (soluble salts)
MERCURY ACETATE
MERCURY FULMINATE
MERCURY NITRATE (acid)
MERCURY OXYCYANIDE
METHYLMERCURY
METHYLMERCURY BORATE
METHYLMERCURY HYDROXIDE
METHYLMERCURY IODIDE
METHYLMERCURY NITRATE
METHYLMERCURY PHOSPHATE
PHENYLMERCURIC ACETATE
PHENYLMERCURY
PHENYLMERCURY OLEATE
TETRABUTYLTIN
TETRAETHYLLEAD
TETRAETHYLTIN
TETRAISOALKYLTINS
TETRAMETHYLLEAD
TETRAPENTYLTIN
TETRAPROPYLTIN
TIN (organic compounds)
TRIBUTYLLEAD*
TRIBUTYLTIN*
TRIETHYLLEAD*
TRIETHYLTIN*
TRIMETHYLLEAD*
TRIMETHYLTIN*
TRIPHENYLTIN*
TRIPROPYLTIN*

*probably dimers

— Always, even IN MILD CASES, notify a physician and inform him of
  - the nature of the substance inhaled and
  - the state of the victim and, if possible, his symptoms.

— Always remove the victim from the contaminated area.

— Never give the victim any alcoholic beverage to drink.

A. If the victim is conscious,

1. Remove him from the contaminated area to a quiet, cool, and well-ventilated area.
2. Lay him on his back.
3. Loosen his collar and belt.
4. Speak reassuringly to him.

B. If the victim is coughing badly,

(in addition to the treatment recommended in A)

5. Make him inhale from a gauze pad soaked with
   - a little ethyl alcohol or
   - a few drops of ether

   CAUTION! These liquids are flammable.
6. If necessary, administer oxygen under low pressure, using a PULMOTOR or similar type of equipment.*

NOTE: Only a physician can treat the victim and will keep him under prolonged medical supervision.

*See Vital Equipment, page 4.

IN CASE OF INHALATION OF

(Alkylaluminum compounds)
ALUMINUM (dust)
ALUMINUM ALKYLS
(Aluminum hydrate)
ALUMINUM HYDROXIDE
ALUMINUM OXIDE
ASBESTOS
CALCIUM CARBONATE
CALCIUM CHLORIDE
CARBON
CARBON BLACK
DIETHYLALUMINUM CHLORIDE
DIETHYLALUMINUM HYDRIDE
DISODIUM PHOSPHATE
KAOLIN
LEAD (metal fumes)
LEAD ACETATE
LEAD ANTIMONATE
LEAD ARSENATE
LEAD CARBONATE
LEAD CHLORIDE
LEAD CHROMATE (red)
LEAD CHROMATE (yellow)
LEAD DIOXIDE
LEAD NITRATE
LEAD OXIDE (PbO)
LEAD OXIDE (red)
LEAD OXYCHLORIDE
LEAD SUBACETATE
LEAD SULFIDE
MAGNESIUM CHLORIDE
MAGNESIUM SULFATE
POLY(VINYL CHLORIDE)
POTASSIUM CHLORIDE
SILICA
SODIUM BICARBONATE
SODIUM CHLORIDE
SODIUM HYPOSULFITE
SODIUM SULFATE
SODIUM THIOCYANATE
SODIUM THIOSULFATE
TALC
THIOCYANATES
TITANIUM (dust)
TITANIUM OXIDE
TRIETHYLALUMINUM
TRIISOBUTYLALUMINUM
TRIMETHYLALUMINUM
TUNGSTEN CARBIDE

— Do not permit the victim to remain in a highly dusty atmosphere without respiratory protection.

---

1. Make the victim blow his nose to remove the dust but discourage him from sniffling.
2. If there is any doubt about the victim's condition, send or escort him to the infirmary, first-aid room, or hospital.

IN CASE OF INHALATION OF DUST OF

ALKALI DICHROMATES (Ca, K, Na)
ALKALI *META*-BORATES (K, Na)
ALUMINUM CHLORIDE
(Aluminum trichloride)
BORIC ACID
CALCIUM CARBIDE
CALCIUM DICHROMATE
CALCIUM HYPOCHLORITE
CALCIUM OXIDE
(Caustic lyes)
CHLORINATED LIME
CHROMIC ACID
CHROMIUM CHLORIDE
COPPER CHLORIDE
COPPER SULFATE
IRON CHLORIDE
(Lime)
PERBORATES (K, Na)
PHTHALIC ANHYDRIDE
POTASSIUM (metal)
POTASSIUM BORATE
POTASSIUM CHROMATE
POTASSIUM DICHROMATE
POTASSIUM FLUOSILICATE
POTASSIUM HYDROXIDE
POTASSIUM OXIDE
SODIUM (metal)
SODIUM BORATE
SODIUM CHROMATE
SODIUM DICHROMATE
SODIUM FLUOSILICATE
SODIUM HYDROXIDE
SODIUM HYPOCHLORITE
SODIUM OXIDE
SODIUM PEROXIDE
TITANIUM CHLORIDES (Tri-, Tetra-)
ZINC CHLORIDE

— Always remove the victim from the contaminated area.

— Notify a physician immediately and inform him of
- the nature of the substance inhaled and
- the state of the victim and, if possible, his symptoms.

— If the victim has any respiratory difficulties, prevent him from unnecessary exertion or movements.

— Never give an unconscious person anything to drink.

A. If the victim's symptoms are limited to prickling in the nose,

1. Make him blow his nose to remove the substance but discourage him from sniffling.

2. If necessary, send the victim to the dispensary, first-aid room, or hospital.

B. If the victim is conscious but has difficulty breathing,

1. Remove him from the contaminated area to a quiet, cool, and well-ventilated area.

2. Lay him down with his legs raised.

3. Loosen his collar and belt.
4. Cover him with a blanket.
5. Speak reassuringly to him.

C. If the victim is coughing badly,

(in addition to the treatment recommended in B)

6. Make him inhale from a gauze pad soaked with
   - a little ethyl alcohol or
   - a few drops of ether.

   } CAUTION! These liquids are flammable.
7. As soon as possible, administer oxygen under low pressure with a PULMOTOR or similar type of equipment.*

D. If the victim's face is blue or pale,

1. Remove him from the contaminated area to a quiet, cool, and well-ventilated area.
2. Lay him **flat on his back** with his head turned to one side and his legs raised.
3. Loosen his collar and belt.
4. Cover him with a blanket.
5. Administer oxygen under low pressure with a PULMOTOR or similar type of equipment.* **Never administer Carbogen** (mixture of oxygen and carbon dioxide).

E. If the victim is unconscious but breathing,

(in addition to the treatment recommended in D)

6. Continue to administer oxygen until the physician arrives.

NOTE: The physician may keep the victim under medical supervision for 1 or 2 days.

*See Vital Equipment, page 4.

IN CASE OF INHALATION OF

ACETONE CYANOHYDRIN
ACRYLONITRILE
BITTER ALMOND ESSENCE
CYANOGEN CHLORIDE
FERRICYANIDES (K, Na)
FERROCYANIDES (K, Na)
HYDROCYANIC ACID
NITROFERRICYANIDES
POTASSIUM CYANIDE
SODIUM CYANIDE

— First aiders must take precautions for their own safety if they must enter the contaminated area to help the victim.

— Always remove the victim from the contaminated area.

— Notify a physician immediately and inform him of
  - the nature of the product inhaled and
  - the state of the victim and, if possible, his symptoms.

— Never give an unconscious person anything to drink.

A. If the victim is conscious,

1. Remove him quickly from the contaminated area to a quiet, cool, and well-ventilated area.
2. Lay him flat on his back.
3. Calm and reassure him.
4. Loosen his collar and belt.
5. Cover him with a blanket.
6. Protect him from injuring himself by convulsive movements.
7. Hold his head back to make breathing easier, if necessary.

B. If the victim is unconscious but still breathing,

(in addition to the treatment indicated in A)

8. Remove dentures or partial plates.
9. Break an ampoule of amyl nitrite (0.2 ml) into a gauze pad or clean cloth and make the victim inhale the vapors for 3 minutes.

10. Repeat this treatment every 5 minutes (maximum 3 ampoules).
11. As soon as possible, administer oxygen under low pressure with a PULMOTOR or similar type of equipment,* if necessary, until the physician arrives.

C. If the victim has stopped breathing,

1. Carry out the treatment in A **very quickly**.
2. Begin artificial respiration **(never mouth-to-mouth resuscitation)** as quickly as possible.
3. As soon as possible, administer oxygen under low pressure with a PULMOTOR or similar type of equipment.*
4. Continue the treatment until he begins to breathe unaided.
5. As soon as he breathes again, remove the oxygen mask.
6. Break an ampoule of amyl nitrite (0.2 ml) into a gauze pad and make him inhale the vapors for 3 minutes.
7. Repeat this treatment every 5 minutes (maximum 3 ampoules).
8. Administer oxygen again until the physician arrives.

*See Vital Equipment, page 4.

First aid **IN CASE OF INGESTION OF**

ACETALDEHYDE
ACETIC ACID
ACETIC ANHYDRIDE
ACROLEIN
ARSENIC (soluble salts)
ARSENIC TRICHLORIDE
BROMINE
BUTYRALDEHYDE
CHLORINE
CHLORINE DIOXIDE
CHLOROACETIC ACID
ETHYL CHLOROFORMATE
FLUORINE
FLUOSILICIC ACID
FORMALDEHYDE
FORMIC ACID
HYDRIODIC ACID
HYDROBROMIC ACID
HYDROCHLORIC ACID
HYDROFLUORIC ACID
(Hydrogen chloride)
HYDROGEN PEROXIDE
IODINE
ISOBUTYRALDEHYDE
METHYL CHLOROFORMATE
NITRIC ACID
OSMIC ACID
OXALIC ACID
PERACETIC ACID
PERCHLORIC ACID
PHENOL
PHOSPHORIC ACID
PHOSPHORUS CHLORIDES
PHOSPHORUS PENTACHLORIDE
PHOSPHORUS TRICHLORIDE
POTASSIUM CHLORITE
POTASSIUM FLUORIDE
POTASSIUM FLUOSILICATE
PROPIONALDEHYDE
SODIUM CHLORITE
SODIUM FLUORIDE
SODIUM FLUOSILICATE
SULFUR DIOXIDE
SULFURIC ACID
SULFUROUS ACID
SULFUR TRIOXIDE
TRICHLOROACETIC ACID

— Never give the victim sodium bicarbonate in powder or solution and never attempt to neutralize the acid with a strong base (ammonia or soda, etc.).

— Never try to make the victim vomit if he has swallowed acid.

— Never give an unconscious person anything to drink.

— In all cases, notify a physician and inform him of
- the nature of the ingested product and
- the state of the victim and, if possible, his symptoms.

A. If the victim is conscious,

1. Remove him from the contaminated area to a quiet, cool, and well-ventilated area where he can rest.

2. Make him rinse his mouth liberally with cold water.

3. Loosen his collar and belt.

4. Never give him water to drink if he has swallowed a strong acid (such as SULFURIC ACID) but give him as much water as he wants if he has swallowed a weak, concentrated acid solution.

5. Except in the case of HYDROGEN PEROXIDE, he can be given either
   - milk (as much as he wants)* or
   - milk of magnesia or
   - milk of lime or
   - calcined magnesia in water or
   - emollients such as table oil or fresh eggs.

6. Lay him down with his legs raised.

7. Cover him with a blanket.

8. Prevent him from moving or speaking unnecessarily.

B. If the victim's face is blue,

1. Lay him down on his back with his head turned to one side.

2. Administer oxygen under low pressure with a PULMOTOR or similar type of equipment† (**never Carbogen** [mixture of oxygen and carbon dioxide]), if necessary, until physician arrives.

*In the case of ingestion of FLUORINE compounds
— Do not let the victim vomit.
— Give him large doses of effervescent calcium gluconate tablets (6 tablets Calciofon, Calglucon, Ebucim, Glucal, or Glubiogen) diluted in copious amounts of fluid (water or milk) to drink.
— Take him to the hospital immediately.

†See Vital Equipment, page 4.

C. If the victim is unconscious but still breathing,

1. Lay him down on his back (except if he is vomiting, when he should lie with his head lowered and turned to one side to prevent him from suffocating).
2. Remove dentures or partial plates.
3. Loosen his collar and belt.
4. Cover him with a blanket.
5. Administer oxygen under low pressure with a PULMOTOR or similar type of equipment* (never use Carbogen [mixture of oxygen and carbon dioxide] if his face is blue), if necessary, until physician arrives.

D. If the victim has stopped breathing,

1. Lay him down and **immediately** begin artificial respiration or mouth-to-mouth resuscitation, or use an AMBU-type bellow.*
2. At the same time, loosen his collar and belt.
3. Cover him with a blanket.
4. Continue artificial respiration with a PULMOTOR or similar type equipment,* administering oxygen under low pressure, until the victim begins to breathe unaided and, if necessary, until the physician arrives.

*See Vital Equipment, page 4.

IN CASE OF INGESTION OF

ALKALI DICHROMATES (Ca, K, Na)
ALKALI *META*-BORATES (K, Na)
ALLYL ALCOHOL
ALLYL CHLORIDE
ALLYL GLYCIDYL ETHER
ALUMINUM CHLORIDE
(Aluminum trichloride)
BORIC ACID
CALCIUM DICHROMATE
CALCIUM HYPOCHLORITE
CHLORINATED LIME
CHROMIC ACID
CHROMIUM CHLORIDE
COPPER CHLORIDE
COPPER SULFATE
DIEPOXYBUTANE
DIGLYCIDYL ETHER
EPICHLOROHYDRIN
ETHYL ACRYLATE
ETHYLENE OXIDE
GLYCIDOL
GLYCIDYL ACRYLATE
IRON CHLORIDE
ISOCYANATES
LEAD (metal fumes)
LEAD ACETATE
LEAD ANTIMONATE
LEAD ARSENATE
LEAD CARBONATE
LEAD CHLORIDE
LEAD CHROMATE (red)
LEAD CHROMATE (yellow)
LEAD DIOXIDE
LEAD NITRATE
LEAD OXIDE (PbO)
LEAD OXIDE (red)
LEAD OXYCHLORIDE
LEAD SUBACETATE
LEAD SULFIDE
MERCURIC CHLORIDE
MERCURIC IODIDE
MERCUROUS CHLORIDE
MERCUROUS IODIDE
MERCURY (metal)
MERCURY (soluble salts)
MERCURY ACETATE
MERCURY NITRATE (acid)
MERCURY OXYCYANIDE
METHYL ACRYLATE
NICKEL (fumes and dust)
NICKEL CARBONYL
PERBORATES (K, Na)
PHTHALIC ANHYDRIDE
POTASSIUM BORATE
POTASSIUM CHROMATE
POTASSIUM DICHROMATE
PROPYLENE OXIDE
SODIUM BORATE
SODIUM CHROMATE
SODIUM DICHROMATE
SODIUM HYPOCHLORITE
STYRENE
TITANIUM CHLORIDES (Tri-, Tetra-)
ZINC CHLORIDE

— Never give an unconscious person anything to drink.

— If the victim turns blue, lay him on his back with his legs raised.

— In every case notify a physician and inform him of
  - the nature of the ingested product and
  - the state of the victim and, if possible, his symptoms.

A. If the victim is conscious,

1. Make him rinse his mouth liberally with cold water.
2. Carry him to a quiet, cool, and well-ventilated area.
3. Sit him down and loosen his collar and belt.
4. Give him plenty of water to drink.
5. Induce vomiting by
   - making him drink a glass of tepid, salted water or
   - asking him to stick his fingers down his throat or
   - tickling his uvula with the handle of a spoon.
6. If possible, give him
   - as much milk as he wants (with a raw egg) or
   - an emollient such as table oil or raw eggs but never alcohol.
7. Cover him with a blanket.
8. If the victim is pale, lay him on his back with his head turned to one side.

B. If the victim is unconscious but still breathing,

1. Lay him down with his trunk raised (if the victim is vomiting uncontrollably, he should lie with his head down and turned to one side to avoid suffocation).
2. Remove dentures or partial plates.
3. Loosen his collar and belt.
4. Cover him with a blanket.
5. Administer oxygen under low pressure with a PULMOTOR or similar type of equipment,* if necessary, until the physician arrives.

NOTE: The physician will keep the victim under medical supervision for at least 2 days.

*See Vital Equipment, page 4.

IN CASE OF INGESTION OF

ALIPHATIC AMINES
AMMONIA
AMMONIUM CARBONATE
AMMONIUM HYDROXIDE
(Ammonia water)
BUTYLAMINES
CALCIUM CARBIDE
CALCIUM HYDROXIDE
CALCIUM OXIDE
(Caustic lyes)
DIBUTYLAMINES
DIETHYLAMINE
DIMETHYLAMINE
DIPROPYLAMINES
ETHYLAMINE
(Lime)
LITHIUM CARBONATE
METHYLAMINE
MILK OF LIME
POTASSIUM (metal)
POTASSIUM CARBONATE
POTASSIUM HYDROXIDE
POTASSIUM OXIDE
PROPYLAMINES
SODIUM (metal)
SODIUM CARBONATE
SODIUM HYDROXIDE
SODIUM OXIDE
SODIUM PEROXIDE
SODIUM SILICATE
TRIETHYLAMINE
TRIMETHYLAMINE
TRISODIUM PHOSPHATE

— Never attempt to neutralize a basic caustic (corrosive) substance with a strong acid, even if diluted.

— Never attempt to make the victim vomit if vomiting is not spontaneous.

— In every case notify a physician and inform him of
- the nature of the ingested product and
- the state of the victim and, if possible, his symptoms.

A. If the victim is conscious,

1. Make him rinse his mouth liberally with cold water.
2. If possible, give him
   - cold water
   - milk with one or two raw eggs
   - fruit juice
   - a glass of vinegar and water (⅓ vinegar—⅔ water).
3. Give him a piece of ice to suck in order to soothe the pain in his mouth.

B. If the victim suffers from shock,

1. Make sure he does not catch cold
2. Lay him down with his head lowered and wrap him in a blanket.

NOTE: The physician will keep the victim under medical supervision for at least 2 days.

IN CASE OF INGESTION OF

BENZENE
CYCLOHEXANE
DECANE
ETHYL ETHER
GASOLINE
HEPTANE
HEXANE
NONANE
OCTANE
PENTANE
PETROLEUM ETHERS
TOLUENE
WHITE SPIRIT
XYLENES

— Do not make the victim vomit even if he is conscious (risk of pulmonary complications).

— Never administer
  - alcohol, milk, fatty foods.

— Never give an unconscious victim anything to drink.

— Even in mild cases, notify a physician and inform him of
  - the nature of the ingested product and
  - the state of the victim and, if possible, his symptoms.

A. If the victim is conscious,

1. Sit or lay him down with his legs raised in a quiet, cool, and well-ventilated area.
2. Make sure he does not catch cold; cover him with a blanket.
3. Give him a tablespoon of mineral oil (Nujol) followed by a glass of water to which a tablespoon of magnesium or sodium sulfate has been added.

B. If the victim is unconscious and has breathing difficulties,

1. Lay him down with his legs raised.
2. Remove dentures or partial plates.
3. Loosen his collar and belt.
4. Cover him with a blanket.

5. Administer oxygen under low pressure with a PULMOTOR or similar type of equipment,* if necessary, until the physician arrives.

C. If the victim is unconscious but still breathing,

1. Lay him flat on his back with his legs raised.
2. Remove dentures or partial plates.
3. Loosen his collar and belt.
4. Cover him with a blanket.
5. Administer oxygen under low pressure with a PULMOTOR or similar type of equipment,* if necessary, until the physician arrives.

D. If the victim has stopped breathing,

1. Lay him down and **immediately** begin artificial respiration or mouth-to-mouth resuscitation.
2. At the same time, loosen his collar and belt.
3. Cover him with a blanket.
4. Continue artificial respiration with a PULMOTOR or similar type of equipment,* administering oxygen under low pressure until he begins to breathe and, if necessary, until the physician arrives.

*See Vital Equipment, page 4.

IN CASE OF INGESTION OF

ACETONE
ALIPHATIC ALCOHOLS
AMYL ACETATE
BUTANOL
BUTYL ACETATE
CARBON TETRACHLORIDE
CHLOROBENZENE
CHLOROETHANES
(Mono-, Di-)
CHLOROETHANES
(Tri-, Tetra-)
CHLOROFORM
CHLOROMETHANES
(Di-, Tri-, Tetra-)
CHLOROPENTAFLUORO-
ETHANE
CHLOROPROPANES
CHLOROPROPENES
CHLORTHION
DDVP
DECANOL
DEMETON
DIAZINON
DICHLOROBENZENES
DICHLOROETHANES
DICHLOROETHYLENES
DICHLOROPROPANES
DICHLOROTETRAFLUORO-
ETHANES
DIETHYLENE GLYCOL
DIISOBUTYLCARBINOL
DIPTEREX
DIPYRIDYL CHLORIDE
DIPYRIDYL DIMETHYL
SULFATE
DIQUAT
EPN
ETHYL ACETATE
ETHYL ALCOHOL
ETHYLENE GLYCOL
ETHYLHEXYL ACETATE
FREON 112, 113, 114, 115
GLYCERIN
(Gramoxon)
HEPTANOL
HEXACHLOROETHANE
HEXANOL
ISOBUTYL ACETATE
ISOPESTOX
ISOPROPYL ACETATE
MALATHION
METHYL ACETATE
METHYL ALCOHOL
(Methylchloroform)
METHYL PARATHION
OMPA
ORGANOPHOSPHORUS
COMPOUNDS
PARAOXON
PARAQUAT
PARATHION
PENTACHLOROETHANE
PENTANOL
PHOSDRIN
PHOSPHORIC ESTERS
PROPYL ACETATE
PROPYL ALCOHOLS
PROPYLENE GYLCOL
QUATERNARY AMMONIUM
COMPOUNDS
RONNEL
SULFOTEPP
TEPP
TETRACHLORODIFLUORO-
ETHANES
TETRACHLOROETHANES
TETRACHLOROETHYLENE
TRICHLOROETHANES
TRICHLOROETHYLENE
TRICHLOROTRIFLUORO-
ETHANES
TRIETHYLENE GLYCOL
TRITHION
VINYL ACETATE
VINYL CHLORIDE
VINYLIDENE CHLORIDE

— Never give an unconscious victim anything to drink.

— Never try to induce vomiting in an unconscious victim.

— In all instances, even in mild cases, notify a physician and inform him of
  - the nature of the ingested product and
  - the state of the victim and, if possible, his symptoms.

— Never administer alcohol, milk, or fatty foods.

— If the victim is pale or in shock, lay him on his back with his head turned to one side to avoid suffocation if he vomits.

A. If the victim is conscious,

1. Sit or lay him down with his legs raised in a quiet, cool, and well-ventilated area.
2. Cover him with a blanket.
3. Induce vomiting by
   - making him drink a glass of tepid, salted water or
   - asking him to stick his fingers down his throat or
   - tickling his uvula with the handle of a spoon.
4. Subsequently administer a tablespoon of mineral oil (Nujol) followed by a glass of water to which a tablespoon of sodium or magnesium sulfate has been added.
5. In case of tiredness give him a cup of strong coffee or tea.

B. If the victim is unconscious and has breathing difficulties,

1. Lay him down
   - with his legs raised, **if his face is red**
   - flat on his back, **if his face is pale.**
2. Remove dentures or partial plates.
3. Loosen his collar and belt.
4. Cover him with a blanket.

5. Administer oxygen under low pressure with a PULMOTOR or similar type of equipment,* if necessary, until the physician arrives.

C. If the victim is no longer breathing,

1. Lay him down and **immediately** begin artificial respiration or mouth-to-mouth resuscitation.
2. At the same time, loosen his collar and belt.
3. Cover him with a blanket.
4. Continue artificial respiration with a PULMOTOR or similar type of equipment,* administering oxygen under low pressure until the victim begins to breathe and, if necessary, until the physician arrives.

The physician will keep the victim under medical supervision for at least 2 days because of the risk of acute pulmonary edema and possible injury to the liver and kidneys.

Do not administer ADRENALINE or EPINEPHRINE to a victim of chlorinated-solvent poisoning.

IN THE CASE OF POISONING BY

— QUATERNARY AMMONIUM COMPOUNDS

— DIPYRIDYL CHLORIDE, DIPYRIDYLDIMETHYL SULFATE, PARAQUAT, Gramoxon, DIQUAT

it would be beneficial to administer an aqueous suspension of fuller's earth (300 g per 1 liter of water) to the victim after he has vomited.

IN CASE OF POISONING BY AN ORGANOPHOSPHORUS COMPOUND

Only a physician is competent to treat the victim so he should be called without delay.

*See Vital Equipment, page 4.

IN CASE OF INGESTION OF

BARIUM (soluble salts)
BARIUM ACETATE
BARIUM CARBONATE
BARIUM CHLORIDE
BARIUM FLUORIDE
BARIUM HYDROXIDE
BARIUM NITRATE
BARIUM OXIDE
BARIUM SULFIDE

— Never give an unconscious person anything to drink.

— In all instances, even in mild cases, notify a physician and inform him of
  - the nature of the ingested product and
  - the state of the victim and, if possible, his symptoms.

A. If the victim is conscious,

1. Sit or lay him in a quiet, cool, and well-ventilated area.
2. Induce vomiting by
   - asking the victim to stick his fingers down his throat or
   - tickling his uvula with the handle of a spoon.
3. Subsequently administer 2 tablespoons of sodium or magnesium sulfate dissolved in water, to convert the soluble barium to insoluble barium sulfate, which is nontoxic.
4. Give him a cup of strong coffee or tea if he is weak or tired.

B. If the victim is unconscious and has breathing difficulties,

1. Lay him on his back if his face is pale.
2. Remove dentures or partial plates.
3. Loosen his collar and belt.
4. Cover him with a blanket.
5. Administer oxygen under low pressure with a PULMOTOR or similar type of equipment,* if necessary, until the physician arrives.

*See Vital Equipment, page 4.

C. If the victim has stopped breathing,

1. Lay him down and **immediately** begin artificial respiration or mouth-to-mouth resuscitation or use an AMBU-type bellows.*
2. At the same time, loosen his collar and belt.
3. Cover him with a blanket.

   In the case of ingestion of BARIUM FLUORIDE,

   — do not let the victim vomit.

   — give him large doses of effervescent calcium gluconate tablets (6 tablets Calciofon, Calglucon, Ebucim, Glucal, or Glubiogen) diluted in copious amounts of fluids (water or milk) to drink.

   — refer him to the hospital.
4. Continue artificial respiration with a PULMOTOR or similar type of equipment,* administering oxygen under low pressure until the victim begins to breathe unaided and, if necessary, until the physician arrives.

*See Vital Equipment, page 4.

IN CASE OF INGESTION OF

ANILINE
CHLORONITROBENZENES
DIMETHYLANILINE
DINITROBENZENES
DINITROCRESOLS
DINITROPHENOLS
DNBP
DNOC
ETHYLENE GLYCOL DINITRATE
ETHYL NITRATE
METHYL NITRATE
NITROANILINES
NITROBENZENE
NITROGLYCERIN
NITROPHENOLS
PENTACHLOROPHENATES
PENTACHLOROPHENOL
PHENYLHYDRAZINE
PHENYLHYDROXYLAMINE
PROPYL NITRATE
TOLUIDINES
TRINITROBENZENE
XYLIDINES

— In all instances, even in mild cases, notify a physician and inform him of
  - the nature of the ingested product and
  - the state of the victim and, if possible, his symptoms.

— If the victim turns blue, lay him on his back with his legs raised.

— Never give an unconscious person anything to drink.

— Do not administer alcohol, milk, eggs, or oil.

A. If the victim is conscious and his face is not blue,

1. Sit or lay him down with his legs raised in a quiet, cool, and well-ventilated area.
2. Cover him with a blanket.
3. Induce vomiting as soon as possible by
   - making him drink a glass of tepid, salted water or
   - asking him to stick his finger down his throat or
   - tickling his uvula with the handle of a spoon.
4. Subsequently administer 1 tablespoon of liquid paraffin.
5. Give him a cup of strong coffee or tea if he is tired.

B. If the victim is conscious and his face is blue,

(in addition to the treatment recommended in A)

6. Lay him flat on his back with his head turned to one side.
7. Make him inhale oxygen under low pressure with a PULMOTOR or similar type of equipment* (**never Carbogen** [mixture of oxygen and carbon dioxide]), if necessary, until the physician arrives.

*See Vital Equipment, page 4.

IN CASE OF INGESTION OF

AMMONIUM CHLORATE
AMMONIUM PERCHLORATE
CALCIUM CHLORIDE
POTASSIUM CHLORATE
POTASSIUM CHLORIDE
POTASSIUM PERCHLORATE
SODIUM BICARBONATE
SODIUM CHLORATE
SODIUM CHLORIDE
SODIUM PERCHLORATE

— Notify a physician who should be informed of
- the nature of the ingested product and
- the state of the victim and, if possible, his symptoms.

---

1. Make the victim vomit by
   - making him drink a glass of tepid, salted water or
   - asking him to stick his finger down his throat or
   - tickling his uvula with the handle of a spoon.
2. Afterwards give him as much milk or water as he wants.

NOTE: If the victim complains of pains in his mouth or stomach, send him to the hospital. The physician should be informed of the nature of the ingested product.

In case of ingestion of perchlorates, the physician will keep the patient under observation for several days, giving special attention to the renal function.

IN CASE OF INGESTION OF

(Alkylmercury compounds)
(Alkyltin compounds)
DIBUTYLLEAD
DIBUTYLTIN
DIETHYLLEAD
DIETHYLMERCURY
DIETHYLTIN
DIHEXYLTIN
DIIODODIETHYLTIN
DIMETHYLMERCURY
DIMETHYLTIN
DIOCTYLTIN
ETHYLMERCURY
ETHYLMERCURIC CHLORIDE
ETHYLMERCURIC HYDROXIDE
LEAD OLEATE
LEAD PHENATE
LEAD PHTHALATE
LEAD STEARATE
MERCURY (organic compounds)
MERCURY FULMINATE
(Mercury phenylacetate)
METHYLMERCURY
METHYLMERCURY BORATE
METHYLMERCURY HYDROXIDE
METHYLMERCURY IODIDE
METHYLMERCURY NITRATE
METHYLMERCURY PHOSPHATE
PHENYLMERCURIC ACETATE
PHENYLMERCURY
PHENYLMERCURY OLEATE
TETRABUTYLTIN
TETRAETHYLLEAD
TETRAETHYLTIN
TETRAISOALKYLTINS
TETRAMETHYLLEAD
TETRAPENTYLTIN
TETRAPROPYLTIN
TIN (organic compounds)
TRIBUTYLLEAD*
TRIBUTYLTIN*
TRIETHYLLEAD*
TRIETHYLTIN*
TRIMETHYLLEAD*
TRIMETHYLTIN*
TRIPHENYLTIN*
TRIPROPYLTIN*

*probably dimers

— In all instances, even mild cases, notify a physician immediately and inform him of
  - the nature of the ingested product and
  - the state of the victim and, if possible, his symptoms.

— Never administer any alcoholic beverage.

— Never give an unconscious person anything to drink.

---

1. Make the victim rinse his mouth copiously with cool water.
2. Sit or lay him down with his legs raised in a quiet, cool, and well-ventilated area.
3. Give him as much water or milk as he wants.

4. Induce vomiting by
   - making him drink a glass of tepid, salted water or
   - asking him to stick his fingers down his throat or
   - tickling his uvula with the handle of a spoon.
5. Cover him with a blanket.

NOTE: Only the physician is competent to treat the victim and will keep him under medical supervision for some time.

IN CASE OF INGESTION OF

ALKANES (liquids and solids)
ALUMINUM (dust)
(Aluminum hydrate)
ALUMINUM HYDROXIDE
ALUMINUM OXIDE
ASBESTOS
CALCIUM CARBONATE
CARBON
CARBON BLACK
CHLORONAPHTHALENES
DIPHENYL
DIPHENYLAMINE
KAOLIN
NAPHTHALENE
NAPHTHYLAMINES
PARAFFINS (solid compounds)
PHENYLNAPHTHYLAMINES
POLY(VINYL CHLORIDE)
SILICA
TALC
TITANIUM (dust)
TITANIUM OXIDE
TUNGSTEN CARBIDE

— Notify a physician and inform him of
- the nature of the ingested product and
- the state of the victim and, if possible, his symptoms.

---

1. Make the victim vomit by
   - making him drink a glass of tepid, salted water or
   - asking him to stick his fingers down his throat or
   - tickling his uvula with the handle of a spoon.
2. Afterwards administer 1 tablespoon of mineral oil (Nujol) or half a glass of peanut oil.

NOTE: Only the physician is competent to treat the victim who has accidentally ingested asbestos.

IN CASE OF INGESTION OF

ACETONE CYANOHYDRIN
ACRYLONITRILE
BITTER ALMOND ESSENCE
CHERRY LAUREL WATER
CYANOGEN CHLORIDE
FERRICYANIDES (K, Na)
FERROCYANIDES (K, Na)
HYDROCYANIC ACID
NITROFERRICYANIDES
POTASSIUM CYANIDE
SODIUM CYANIDE
THIOCYANATES

— In all instances, **even in mild cases**, notify a physician who should be informed of
  - the nature of the ingested product and
  - the state of the victim and, if possible, his symptoms.

— Never give an unconscious person anything to drink.

A. If the victim is conscious but excited,

1. Sit him down.
2. Reassure him and try to calm him.
3. Loosen his collar and belt.
4. Induce vomiting by
   - asking him to stick his fingers down his throat, or
   - tickling his uvula with the handle of a spoon.
5. Give him a large glass of water to which thiosulfate (sodium hyposulfite) has been added (1% solution).

B. If the victim is unconscious but still breathing,

1. Lay him flat on his back.
2. Remove dentures or partial plates.
3. Loosen his collar and belt.
4. Cover him with a blanket.
5. Break a 0.2 ml ampoule of amyl nitrite into a gauze pad and make the victim inhale the vapors for 3 minutes.

6. Repeat this treatment every 5 minutes (maximum 3 ampoules).
7. Protect him from injuring himself by convulsive movements.
8. Keep his head bent backwards to help him breathe.
9. As soon as possible, administer oxygen under low pressure with a PULMOTOR or similar type of equipment,* if necessary, until the physician arrives.

C. If the victim has stopped breathing,

1. Lay him flat on his back.
2. Quickly loosen his collar and belt.
3. Immediately begin artificial respiration (never use mouth-to-mouth resuscitation).
4. As soon as possible, administer oxygen under low pressure with a PULMOTOR or similar type of equipment.*
5. Continue the treatment until the physician arrives or until the victim breathes unaided.
6. As soon as the victim is breathing again, remove the oxygen mask.
7. Break a 0.2 ml ampoule of amyl nitrite into a gauze pad and make the victim inhale the vapor for 3 minutes.
8. Repeat this treatment every 5 minutes (maximum 3 ampoules).
9. Afterwards administer oxygen again until the physician arrives.

*See Vital Equipment, page 4.

First aid **IN CASE OF SKIN CONTACT WITH**

ACETALDEHYDE
ACETIC ACID
ACETIC ANHYDRIDE
ACROLEIN
ARSENIC TRICHLORIDE
ARSINE (gas)
BROMINE
BUTYRALDEHYDE
CHLORINE
CHLORINE DIOXIDE
CHLOROACETIC ACID
ETHYL CHLOROFORMATE
FORMALDEHYDE
FORMIC ACID
HYDRIODIC ACID
HYDROBROMIC ACID
HYDROCHLORIC ACID
(Hydrogen chloride)
HYDROGEN PEROXIDE
HYDROGEN SELENIDE
HYDROGEN SULFIDE
IODINE
ISOBUTYRALDEHYDE
METHYL CHLOROFORMATE
NITRIC ACID
OSMIC ACID
OXALIC ACID
OZONE
PERACETIC ACID
PERCHLORIC ACID
PHENOL
PHOSGENE
PHOSPHINE
PHOSPHORIC ACID
PHOSPHORUS CHLORIDES
PHOSPHORUS PENTACHLORIDE
PHOSPHORUS TRICHLORIDE
POTASSIUM CHLORITE
PROPIONALDEHYDE
SODIUM CHLORITE
SULFUR DIOXIDE
SULFURIC ACID
SULFUROUS ACID
SULFUR TRIOXIDE
TRICHLOROACETIC ACID

— It is vital to apply first aid without delay.

— In the case of extensive splashing of the product, wash the victim down under a cold or luke-warm shower or a hand-held hose, at the same time protecting his eyes.

— First aiders must take precautions for their own safety when handling contaminated clothing.

— Notify a physician and inform him of the nature of the substance and the accident.

— Without medical advice, never apply an oily substance to the affected area.

---

1. Remove the victim from the source of contamination and take him **immediately** to the nearest shower.
2. Remove clothing from the affected areas as quickly as possible (cutting it off if necessary).

3. Wipe off excess chemical **very gently and without delay**.
4. Wash affected area under the shower with mild soap.
5. Dust affected area with powdered sodium bicarbonate.
6. Wash affected area again under the shower with mild soap.
7. Rinse affected area with tepid water.
8. Dry the skin very gently with a clean, soft towel.

In case of burns (inflammation, blisters, or lesions) and in the absence of the physician

9. Apply a dry sterile dressing.
10. Dress the victim in clean clothes or cover him with blankets.
11. Take him to the hospital.

If the victim is in a state of shock,

12. Cover him with a blanket.
13. Carry him on a stretcher, lying on his back.

IN CASE OF SKIN CONTACT WITH

ALKALI DICHROMATES (Ca, K, Na)
ALKALI *META*-BORATES (K, Na)
(Alkylmercury compounds)
(Alkyltin compounds)
ALUMINUM CHLORIDE
(Aluminum trichloride)
AMMONIUM CHLORATE
AMMONIUM PERCHLORATE
ARSENIC (soluble salts)
BARIUM (soluble salts)
BARIUM ACETATE
BARIUM CARBONATE
BARIUM CHLORIDE
BARIUM FLUORIDE
BARIUM HYDROXIDE
BARIUM NITRATE
BARIUM OXIDE
BARIUM SULFIDE
BORIC ACID
CALCIUM CHLORIDE
CALCIUM DICHROMATE
CALCIUM HYPOCHLORITE
CHLORINATED LIME
CHROMIC ACID
CHROMIUM CHLORIDE
COPPER CHLORIDE
COPPER SULFATE
DIBUTYLTIN
DIETHYLMERCURY
DIETHYLTIN
DIHEXYLTIN
DIIODODIETHYLTIN
DIMETHYLMERCURY
DIMETHYLTIN
DIOCTYLTIN
ETHYLMERCURY
ETHYLMERCURIC CHLORIDE
ETHYLMERCURIC HYDROXIDE
IRON CHLORIDE
LEAD ACETATE
LEAD ANTIMONATE
LEAD ARSENATE
LEAD CARBONATE
LEAD CHLORIDE
LEAD CHROMATE (red)
LEAD CHROMATE (yellow)
LEAD DIOXIDE
LEAD NITRATE
LEAD OXIDE (PbO)
LEAD OXIDE (red)
LEAD OXYCHLORIDE
LEAD SUBACETATE
LEAD SULFIDE
MERCURIC CHLORIDE
MERCURIC IODIDE
MERCUROUS CHLORIDE
MERCUROUS IODIDE
MERCURY (metal)
MERCURY (organic compounds)
MERCURY (soluble salts)
MERCURY ACETATE
MERCURY FULMINATE
MERCURY NITRATE (acid)
MERCURY OXYCYANIDE
METHYLMERCURY
METHYLMERCURY BORATE
METHYLMERCURY HYDROXIDE
METHYLMERCURY IODIDE
METHYLMERCURY NITRATE
METHYLMERCURY PHOSPHATE
PERBORATES (K, Na)
PHENYLMERCURIC ACETATE
PHENYLMERCURIC OLEATE
PHENYLMERCURY
PHTHALIC ANHYDRIDE
POTASSIUM BORATE
POTASSIUM CHLORATE
POTASSIUM CHLORIDE
POTASSIUM CHROMATE
POTASSIUM DICHROMATE
POTASSIUM PERCHLORATE
SODIUM BICARBONATE
SODIUM BORATE

SODIUM CHLORATE
SODIUM CHLORIDE
SODIUM CHROMATE
SODIUM DICHROMATE
SODIUM HYPOCHLORITE
SODIUM PERCHLORATE
TETRABUTYLTIN
TRIBUTYLTIN*
TETRAETHYLTIN
TETRAISOALKYLTINS
TETRAPENTYLTIN
TETRAPROPYLTIN
TIN (organic compounds)
TITANIUM CHLORIDES (Tri-, Tetra-)
TRIETHYLTIN*
TRIMETHYLTIN*
TRIPHENYLTIN*
TRIPROPYLTIN*
ZINC CHLORIDE

*probably dimers

— Prevent the substance from corroding moist skin.

— Never apply an oily substance to affected areas without medical advice.

— Notify a physician and inform him of the nature of the chemical and of the accident.

---

1. Remove the victim from source of contamination.
2. Remove clothing from affected area.
3. Wash affected area under the shower.
4. Rinse carefully.
5. Dry gently with a clean, soft towel.

If the skin is inflamed or painful,

6. Contact the medical service, who will treat it in the same way as a heat or thermal burn.
7. Dress the victim in clean clothes.

IN CASE OF SKIN CONTACT WITH

FLUORINE
FLUOSILICIC ACID
HYDROFLUORIC ACID
POTASSIUM FLUORIDE
POTASSIUM FLUOSILICATE
SODIUM FLUORIDE
SODIUM FLUOSILICATE

— It is vital to apply first aid without delay.

— In the case of extensive splashing of the substance, wash the victim down under a cold shower or a hand-held hose, at the same time protecting his eyes.

— First aiders must take precautions for their own safety when handling contaminated clothing.

— Notify a physician and inform him of the nature of the chemical and of the accident.

— Never apply an oily substance on affected areas without medical advice.

---

1. Remove the victim from the source of contamination and take him **immediately** to the nearest shower.
2. First aiders, wearing rubber gloves and air-tight safety goggles, should remove the clothing from affected area under the shower (clothing can be cut away, if necessary). Care should be taken not to contaminate healthy skin or eyes. If the victim is already wearing air-tight safety goggles, do not remove them.
3. Wash him down with cold water for 15 minutes or longer.
4. Dry the skin very gently with a clean, soft towel.
5. Apply calcium gluconate gel 2.5% on the affected skin.
6. Massage the gel **gently** into every burnt area with clean fingers.
7. Dress the victim in clean clothes.

In the case of burns (inflammation, blisters, or painful lesions) and in the absence of a physician,

8. If there is no calcium gluconate gel on hand, rub a clean cube of ice on the painful areas and apply a dry, sterile dressing.

9. Take the victim, wrapped in a blanket, to the hospital as soon as possible.

If the victim shows signs of shock,

10. Cover him with a blanket.
11. Make him lie down in a quiet place on his back with his head down and legs raised until the physician arrives.

NOTE: Oral administration of 6 tablets of effervescent calcium gluconate (Calciofon, Calglucon, Ebucim, Glucal, and Glubiogen tablets) dissolved in water is recommended in case of large burns.

IN CASE OF SKIN CONTACT WITH

ALIPHATIC AMINES
AMMONIA
AMMONIUM HYDROXIDE
(Ammonia water)
BUTYLAMINES
CALCIUM CARBIDE
CALCIUM OXIDE
(Caustic lyes)
DIBUTYLAMINES
DIETHYLAMINE
DIMETHYLAMINE
DIPROPYLAMINES
ETHYLAMINE
(Lime)
METHYLAMINE
POTASSIUM (metal)
POTASSIUM HYDROXIDE
POTASSIUM OXIDE
PROPYLAMINES
SODIUM (metal)
SODIUM HYDROXIDE
SODIUM OXIDE
SODIUM PEROXIDE
TRIETHYLAMINE
TRIMETHYLAMINE

— It is vital to apply first aid without delay.

— In the case of extensive splashing of the substance, wash the victim down under a cold shower or a hand-held hose, at the same time protecting his eyes.

— First aiders must take precautions for their own safety when handling contaminated clothing.

— Notify a physician and inform him of the nature of the chemical and the accident.

— Never apply an oily substance to the affected areas without medical advice.

---

1. Remove the victim from the source of contamination and take him **immediately** to the nearest shower.
2. The first aiders, wearing rubber gloves and air-tight safety goggles, should remove the clothing from the affected areas under the shower (clothing can be cut away, if necessary). Care should be taken not to contaminate healthy skin or eyes. If the victim is already wearing air-tight safety goggles, do not remove them.
3. Continue to wash him down until the feeling of stickiness caused by the caustic (corrosive) substance disappears (for more than an hour, if necessary).
4. Rinse the skin and dry it very gently with a clean, soft towel.

If the skin is inflamed, painful, or shows blisters or lesions,

5. Apply a dry, sterile dressing.
6. Dress the victim in clean clothes or wrap him in a blanket.
7. Take him to the hospital.

If the victim shows signs of shock,

8. Keep him warm.
9. Make him lie down in a quiet place on his back with his head down and legs raised until the physician arrives.

IN CASE OF SKIN CONTACT WITH

ACETYLENE (pure material)
ALKANES (as liquids)
BUTADIENE
BUTANE
CARBON DIOXIDE
CARBON DIOXIDE SNOW
CHLORODIFLUOROETHANE
CHLORODIFLUOROMETHANE
CHLOROETHANES (Mono-, Di-)
CHLOROFLUOROETHANES
CHLOROFLUOROMETHANES
CHLOROMETHANES (Mono-, Di-)
CHLOROTRIFLUORO-ETHYLENE
CHLOROTRIFLUORO-METHANE
DICHLORODIFLUORO-METHANE
DICHLOROETHANES
DICHLOROFLUORO-METHANE
DIFLUOROETHANES
DIFLUOROETHYLENES
(Difluoromethane)
ETHANE (liquid)
ETHYLENE (liquid)
ETHYL ETHER
ETHYL FLUORIDE
FLUOROMETHANE
FREON 11, 12, 13, 14, 21, 22, 116, 142b, 143, 151a, 152a
HEXAFLUOROETHANE
METHANE (liquid)
METHYL CHLORIDE
METHYLENE CHLORIDE
METHYLENE FLUORIDE
NITROGEN (liquid)
PROPANE (as liquid)
PROPYLENE
TETRAFLUOROETHYLENE
TETRAFLUOROMETHANE
TRICHLOROFLUORO-METHANE
TRIFLUOROETHANES
TRIFLUOROMETHANE
VINYL CHLORIDE
VINYL FLUORIDE
VINYLIDENE CHLORIDE
VINYLIDENE FLUORIDE

— If splashes of the chemical have caused freezing of the skin, never rinse the affected area with hot or tepid water.

— Bear in mind the risk of poisoning by vapors released in small rooms.

— Bear in mind the risk of fire and explosion that can be caused by vapors of the chemical when contaminated clothes are dried.

— Prevent liquid products from corroding the skin.

---

1. Remove the victim from the source of contamination.
2. Remove clothing from affected area.
3. Wash affected area with cold water and soap, if necessary, under the shower.

4. Dry carefully with a clean, soft towel.

If the skin is inflamed or painful (freezing),

5. Contact the medical service who will treat it in the same way as a heat or thermal burn.

If the skin is neither inflamed nor painful but simply dry,

6. Apply a little lanolin ointment to the affected area.
7. Get dry, clean clothes for the victim.

IN CASE OF SKIN CONTACT WITH

ACETONE
ALIPHATIC ALCOHOLS
ALLYL ALCOHOL
ALLYL CHLORIDE
ALLYL GLYCIDYL ETHER
AMYL ACETATE
ANILINE
BENZENE
BUTANOL
BUTYL ACETATE
CARBON TETRACHLORIDE
CHLOROBENZENE
CHLOROETHANES (Tri-, Tetra-)
CHLOROFORM
CHLOROMETHANES (Tri-, Tetra-)
CHLORONITROBENZENES
CHLOROPENTAFLUOROETHANE
CHLOROPROPANES
CHLOROPROPENES
CYCLOHEXANE
DECANE
DECANOL
DIBUTYLLEAD
DICHLOROBENZENES
DICHLOROETHYLENES
DICHLOROPROPANES
DICHLOROTETRAFLUOROETHANES
DIEPOXYBUTANE
DIETHYLENE GLYCOL
DIETHYLLEAD
DIGLYCIDYL ETHER
DIISOBUTYLCARBINOL
DIMETHYLANILINE
DINITROBENZENES
DINITROCRESOLS
DINITROPHENOLS
DIPYRIDYL CHLORIDE
DIPYRIDYL DIMETHYL SULFATE
DIQUAT
DNBP
DNOC
EPICHLOROHYDRIN
ETHYL ACETATE
ETHYL ACRYLATE
ETHYL ALCOHOL
ETHYLENE GLYCOL
ETHYLENE GLYCOL DINITRATE
ETHYLENE OXIDE
ETHYLHEXYL ACETATE
ETHYL NITRATE
FREON 112, 113, 114, 115
GASOLINE
GLYCERIN
GLYCIDOL
GLYCIDYL ACRYLATE
(Gramoxon)
HEPTANE
HEPTANOL
HEXACHLOROETHANE
HEXANE
HEXANOL
ISOBUTYL ACETATE
ISOCYANATES
ISOPROPYL ACETATE
LEAD OLEATE
LEAD PHENATE
LEAD PHTHALATE
LEAD STEARATE
METHYL ACETATE
METHYL ACRYLATE
METHYL ALCOHOL
(Methylchloroform)
METHYL NITRATE
NICKEL (dust)
NICKEL CARBONYL
NITROANILINES
NITROBENZENE
NITROGLYCERIN
NITROPHENOLS
NONANE
OCTANE
PARAQUAT
PENTACHLOROETHANE
PENTACHLOROPHENATES
PENTACHLOROPHENOL

PENTANE
PENTANOL
PETROLEUM ETHERS
PHENYLHYDRAZINE
PHENYLHYDROXYLAMINE
PROPYL ACETATE
PROPYL ALCOHOLS
PROPYLENE GLYCOL
PROPYLENE OXIDE
PROPYL NITRATE
QUATERNARY AMMONIUM COMPOUNDS
STYRENE
TETRACHLORODIFLUORO-ETHANES
TETRACHLOROETHANES
TETRACHLOROETHYLENE
TETRAETHYLLEAD
TETRAMETHYLLEAD
TOLUENE
TOLUIDINES
TRIBUTYLLEAD*
TRICHLOROETHANES
TRICHLOROETHYLENE
TRICHLOROTRIFLUORO-ETHANES
TRIETHYLENE GLYCOL
TRIETHYLLEAD*
TRIMETHYLLEAD*
TRINITROBENZENE
VINYL ACETATE
WHITE SPIRIT
XYLENES
XYLIDINES

*probably dimers

— Bear in mind the risk of poisoning by vapors released in small rooms.

— Bear in mind the risk of fire and explosion that may be caused by vapors of the chemical when contaminated clothes are dried.

— Prevent the liquid product from corroding the skin.

---

1. Remove the victim from the source of contamination.
2. Remove clothing from affected area.
3. Wash the skin with soap and water under a shower, if necessary.
4. Dry carefully with a clean, soft towel.

If the skin is inflamed, painful, or blistered,

5. Contact the medical service who will treat it in the same way as a heat or thermal burn.

If the skin is neither red nor painful but simply dry,

6. Apply a little lanolin ointment.
7. Get clean, dry clothes for the victim.

IN THE CASE OF SKIN CONTACT WITH

ALUMINUM (dust)
(Aluminum hydrate)
ALUMINUM HYDROXIDE
ALUMINUM OXIDE
ASBESTOS
CALCIUM CARBONATE
CARBON
CARBON BLACK
DISODIUM PHOSPHATE
KAOLIN
MAGNESIUM CHLORIDE
MAGNESIUM SULFATE
POLY(VINYL CHLORIDE)
SILICA
SODIUM SULFATE
SODIUM THIOSULFATE
TALC
TITANIUM (dust)
TITANIUM OXIDE
TUNGSTEN CARBIDE

1. Remove the victim from the source of contamination.
2. Remove contaminated clothing, if necessary.
3. Wash affected areas with soap and water.
4. Rinse carefully.
5. Dry.
6. Get clean, dry clothes for the victim.

IN CASE OF SKIN CONTACT WITH

ACETONE CYANOHYDRIN
ACRYLONITRILE
BITTER ALMOND ESSENCE
CHERRY LAUREL WATER
CYANOGEN CHLORIDE
FERRICYANIDES (K, Na)
FERROCYANIDES (K, Na)
HYDROCYANIC ACID
NITROFERRICYANIDES
POTASSIUM CYANIDE
SODIUM CYANIDE
SODIUM THIOCYANATE
THIOSULFATES

— Notify a physician and inform him of
  - the nature of the chemical and the accident and
  - the state of the victim and, if possible, his symptoms.

— First aiders must take precautions for their own safety when rescuing a person in a contaminated area.

---

1. Remove the victim from the source of contamination.
2. Remove clothing from affected area as quickly as possible under the shower (clothing may be cut away, if necessary).
3. Remove clothes to prevent the inhalation of toxic vapors that may be released.
4. Wash the victim with soap and water.
5. Rinse carefully.
6. Dry carefully with a clean, soft towel.
7. In every case, send the victim to the hospital.

If the skin is inflamed and painful (ACRYLONITRILE),

8. Apply a dry dressing or, better,
9. Contact the medical service, who will treat it in the same way as a heat or thermal burn.

IN CASE OF SKIN CONTACT WITH

ALKANES (liquids and solids)
AMMONIUM CARBONATE
CALCIUM HYDROXIDE
CHLORONAPHTHALENES
DIPHENYL
DIPHENYLAMINE
LITHIUM CARBONATE
MILK OF LIME
NAPHTHALENE
NAPHTHYLAMINES
PHENYLNAPHTHYLAMINES
POTASSIUM CARBONATE
SODIUM CARBONATE
SODIUM SILICATE
TRISODIUM PHOSPHATE

— Prevent the product from corroding moist skin.

— Never apply an oily substance to affected areas without medical advice.

— Notify a physician and inform him of the nature of the chemical and of the accident.

---

1. Remove the victim from the source of contamination.
2. Remove clothing from affected areas.
3. Wash affected areas with running water; DO NOT USE SOAP.
4. Rinse carefully.
5. Dry gently with a clean, soft towel.

If the skin is inflamed or painful,

6. Contact the medical service, who will treat it in the same way as a heat or thermal burn.
7. Get clean, dry clothes for the victim.

IN CASE OF SKIN CONTACT WITH

(Alkylaluminum compounds)
ALUMINUM ALKYLS
DIETHYLALUMINUM CHLORIDE
DIETHYLALUMINUM HYDRIDE
TRIETHYLALUMINUM
TRIISOBUTYLALUMINUM
TRIMETHYLALUMINUM

— Notify the physician without delay and inform him of the nature of the accident and the urgency of the case.

— Never touch the victim with bare hands.

— Never handle contaminated articles with bare hands.

— Always let blazing articles burn in the open air.

1. Make the victim lie on the ground.
2. **Very quickly and without touching the victim**, wash him down with cold water from a hand-held hose, as if to flush away the chemical* (in other words, do not spray him from the front).
3. Lay the victim flat on his back on a stretcher without removing the burnt clothing.
4. Cover him with a blanket.
5. Take him to the hospital immediately.

*The flames will become more intense when washing begins, but will then die out.

IN CASE OF SKIN CONTACT WITH

CHLORTHION
DDVP
DEMETON
DIAZINON
DIPTEREX
EPN
ISOPESTOX
MALATHION
METHYL PARATHION
OMPA
ORGANOPHOSPHORUS COMPOUNDS
PARAOXON
PARATHION
PHOSDRIN
PHOSPHORIC ESTERS
RONNEL
SULFOTEPP
TEPP
TRITHION

— It is vital to apply first aid without delay.

— In the case of extensive splashing of the chemical, wash the victim down under a cold shower or a hand-held hose.

— First aiders must take precautions for their own safety when handling contaminated clothing.

— Immediately notify a physician and inform him of the nature of the chemical and of the accident.

— Never apply an oily substance to the affected areas without medical advice.

---

1. Remove the victim from the source of contamination and take him **immediately** to the nearest shower.
2. First aiders, wearing rubber gloves and air-tight safety goggles, should remove the clothing from the affected areas under the shower (clothing may be cut away, if necessary). Care should be taken not to contaminate healthy skin or eyes.
3. If the victim is already wearing air-tight safety goggles, do not remove them.

If the victim is conscious but has difficulty in breathing,

1. Lay him on his back with his head down and legs raised.
2. Loosen his collar and belt.
3. Cover him with a blanket.
4. Make him inhale oxygen until the physician arrives.

The physician **should be called immediately to treat the victim.**

First aid **IN CASE OF EYE CONTACT WITH**

ACETALDEHYDE
ACETIC ACID
ACETIC ANHYDRIDE
ACROLEIN
ARSENIC TRICHLORIDE
ARSINE (gas)
BROMINE
BUTYRALDEHYDE
CHLORINE
CHLORINE DIOXIDE
CHLOROACETIC ACID
ETHYL CHLOROFORMATE
FLUORINE
FLUOSILICIC ACID
FORMALDEHYDE
FORMIC ACID
HYDRIODIC ACID
HYDROBROMIC ACID
HYDROCHLORIC ACID
HYDROFLUORIC ACID
(Hydrogen chloride)
HYDROGEN PEROXIDE
HYDROGEN SELENIDE
HYDROGEN SULFIDE
IODINE
ISOBUTYRALDEHYDE
METHYL CHLOROFORMATE
NITRIC ACID
OSMIC ACID
OXALIC ACID
OZONE
PERACETIC ACID
PERCHLORIC ACID
PHENOL
PHOSGENE
PHOSPHINE
PHOSPHORIC ACID
PHOSPHORUS CHLORIDES
PHOSPHORUS PENTACHLORIDE
PHOSPHORUS TRICHLORIDE
POTASSIUM CHLORITE
POTASSIUM FLUORIDE
POTASSIUM FLUOSILICATE
PROPIONALDEHYDE
SODIUM CHLORITE
SODIUM FLUORIDE
SODIUM FLUOSILICATE
SULFUR DIOXIDE
SULFURIC ACID
SULFUROUS ACID
SULFUR TRIOXIDE
TRICHLOROACETIC ACID

— It is imperative to bathe eyes as soon as possible.

— Never introduce oil or ointment into the eyes without medical advice.

— Notify a physician and inform him of the
- name of the chemical and
- nature of the accident.

---

1. Remove the victim from the source of contamination and take him to the nearest eye wash or shower.

2. Immediately wipe away any excess of the chemical (liquid or powder) **very gently** and quickly.

3. Wash affected eye or eyes under slowly running water for 15 minutes or longer, making sure that the victim's eyelids are held wide apart and he moves his eyes slowly in every direction.
4. If great pain persists after washing, the nurse can put 1 or 2 drops of anaesthetizing eye salve, or better still, 1 drop of BENOXINATE (NOVESINE) at 0.4%, into the eye.*
5. If the pain persists, repeat washing the eye for 15 minutes or until the pain is relieved or the pH of the eye returns to normal (touch the white of the eye with litmus paper).

NOTE: The medical service will refer the victim to an ophthalmologist and inform him of the nature of the accident and the chemical.

*In case of splashing of fluorine compounds, especially FLUORINE itself, several drops of sterile calcium gluconate 10% solution (SANDOZ or equivalent) in the eye is highly recommended after washing.

IN CASE OF EYE CONTACT WITH

ALIPHATIC AMINES
AMMONIA
AMMONIUM HYDROXIDE
(Ammonia water)
BUTYLAMINES
CALCIUM CARBIDE
CALCIUM OXIDE
(Caustic lyes)
DIBUTYLAMINES
DIETHYLAMINE
DIMETHYLAMINE
DIPROPYLAMINES
ETHYLAMINE
(Lime)
METHYLAMINE
MILK OF LIME
POTASSIUM (metal)
POTASSIUM HYDROXIDE
POTASSIUM OXIDE
PROPYLAMINES
SODIUM (metal)
SODIUM HYDROXIDE
SODIUM OXIDE
SODIUM PEROXIDE
TRIETHYLAMINE
TRIMETHYLAMINE

— It is imperative to bathe the eyes as soon as possible.

— Never introduce oil or ointment into the eyes without medical advice.

— Notify a physician and inform him of the
- name of the chemical and
- nature of the accident.

---

1. Remove the victim from the source of contamination and take him to the nearest eye wash or shower.
2. Immediately wipe away any excess of the chemical (liquid or powder) **very gently** and quickly.
3. Wash the affected eye or eyes under slowly running water for 15 minutes or longer, making sure that the victim's eyelids are held wide apart and he moves his eyes slowly in every direction.
4. If great pain persists after washing, the nurse can put 1 or 2 drops of anaesthetizing eye salve, or better still, 1 drop of BENOXINATE (NOVESINE) at 0.4%, into the eye.
5. If pain persists, repeat washing the eye **for 2 hours** exactly as described in 3.
6. Check during the treatment that no solid particles of the chemical

remain in the creases of the eye; if they do, continue to wash the eye.

NOTE: The medical service will refer the victim to an ophthalmologist and inform him of the nature of the accident and of the chemical.

IN CASE OF EYE CONTACT WITH

AMMONIUM CARBONATE
ANILINE
CALCIUM HYDROXIDE
CHLORONITROBENZENES
DIMETHYLANILINE
DINITROBENZENES
DINITROCRESOLS
DINITROPHENOLS
DNBP
DNOC
ETHYLENE GLYCOL DINITRATE
ETHYL NITRATE
LITHIUM CARBONATE
METHYL NITRATE
NITROANILINES
NITROBENZENE
NITROGLYCERIN
NITROPHENOLS
PENTACHLOROPHENATES
PENTACHLOROPHENOL
PHENYLHYDRAZINE
PHENYLHYDROXYLAMINE
POTASSIUM CARBONATE
PROPYL NITRATE
SODIUM CARBONATE
SODIUM SILICATE
TOLUIDINES
TRINITROBENZENE
TRISODIUM PHOSPHATE
XYLIDINES

— It is imperative to bathe the eyes as soon as possible.

— Never introduce oil or ointment into the eyes without medical advice.

— Notify a physician and inform him of the
- name of the chemical and
- nature of the accident.

---

1. Remove the victim from the source of contamination and take him to the nearest eye wash or shower.
2. Immediately wash the affected eye or eyes under slowly running water for 15 minutes or longer, making sure that the victim's eyelids are held wide apart and he moves his eyes slowly in every direction.
3. If great pain persists after washing, the nurse can put 1 or 2 drops of anaesthetizing eye salve, or better still, BENOXINATE (NOVESINE) at 0.4%, into the eye.
4. If pain persists, repeat washing the eye for 15 minutes or until the pH of the eye returns to normal (touch the white of the eye with litmus paper).
5. Make sure that no solid particles of the chemical remain in the creases of the eye; if they do, continue to wash the eye.

NOTE: The medical service will refer the victim to an ophthalmologist and inform him of the nature of the accident and of the chemical.

IN CASE OF SPLASHING IN EYES WITH LIQUID PRODUCTS

ACETYLENE (pure material)
ALKANES (as liquids)
BUTADIENE
BUTANE
CARBON DIOXIDE
CARBON DIOXIDE SNOW
CHLORODIFLUOROETHANE
CHLORODIFLUORO-METHANE
CHLOROETHANES (Mono-, Di-)
CHLOROFLUOROETHANES
CHLOROFLUOROMETHANES
CHLOROMETHANES (Mono-, Di-)
CHLOROTRIFLUORO-ETHYLENE
CHLOROTRIFLUORO-METHANE
DICHLORODIFLUORO-METHANE
DICHLOROETHANES
DICHLOROFLUORO-METHANE
DIFLUOROETHANES
DIFLUOROETHYLENES
DIFLUOROMETHANE
ETHANE
ETHYLENE
ETHYL ETHER
ETHYL FLUORIDE
FLUOROMETHANE
FREON 11, 12, 13, 14, 21, 22, 116, 142b, 143, 151a, 152a
HEXAFLUOROETHANE
METHANE
METHYL CHLORIDE
METHYLENE CHLORIDE
METHYLENE FLUORIDE
NITROGEN
PROPANE
PROPENE
(Propylene)
TETRAFLUOROETHYLENE
TETRAFLUOROMETHANE
TRICHLOROFLUORO-METHANE
TRIFLUOROETHANES
TRIFLUOROMETHANE
VINYL CHLORIDE
VINYL FLUORIDE
VINYLIDENE CHLORIDE
VINYLIDENE FLUORIDE

— Never introduce oil or ointment into the eye without medical advice.

— In case of freezing by highly volatile products, never wash the eyes with hot or even tepid water.

— Notify a physician and inform him of the
- name of the chemical and
- nature of the accident.

---

1. Remove the victim from the source of contamination.
2. Open his eyelids wide to let the product evaporate.
3. If the pain persists, the medical service will refer the victim to an

ophthalmologist and inform him of the nature of the accident and the name of the chemical.

4. If the victim cannot tolerate light, protect his eyes with a bandage or handkerchief.

IN CASE OF EYE CONTACT WITH

ACETONE
ACETONE CYANOHYDRIN
ACRYLONITRILE
ALIPHATIC ALCOHOLS
ALLYL ALCOHOL
ALLYL CHLORIDE
ALLYL GLYCIDYL ETHER
AMYL ACETATE
BENZENE
BITTER ALMOND ESSENCE
BUTANOL
BUTYL ACETATE
CARBON TETRACHLORIDE
CHERRY LAUREL WATER
CHLOROBENZENE
CHLOROETHANES (Tri-, Tetra-)
CHLOROFORM
CHLOROMETHANE (Tri-, Tetra-)
CHLOROPENTAFLUORO-ETHANE
CHLOROPROPANES
CHLOROPROPENES
CYANOGEN CHLORIDE
CYCLOHEXANE
DECANE
DECANOL
DICHLOROBENZENES
DICHLOROETHYLENES
DICHLOROPROPANES
DICHLOROTETRAFLUORO-ETHANES
DIEPOXYBUTANE
DIETHYLENE GLYCOL
DIGLYCIDYL ETHER
DIISOBUTYLCARBINOL
DIPYRIDYL CHLORIDE
DIPYRIDYL DIMETHYL SULFATE
DIQUAT
EPICHLOROHYDRIN
ETHYL ACETATE
ETHYL ACRYLATE
ETHYL ALCOHOL
ETHYLENE GLYCOL
ETHYLENE OXIDE
ETHYLHEXYL ACETATE
FERRICYANIDES (K, Na)
FERROCYANIDES (K, Na)
FREON 112, 113, 114, 115
GASOLINE
GLYCERIN
GLYCIDOL
GLYCIDYL ACRYLATE
(Gramoxon)
HEPTANE
HEPTANOL
HEXACHLOROETHANE
HEXANE
HEXANOL
HYDROCYANIC ACID
ISOBUTYL ACETATE
ISOCYANATES
ISOPROPYL ACETATE
METHYL ACETATE
METHYL ACRYLATE
METHYL ALCOHOL
(Methylchloroform)
NICKEL (fumes and dust)
NICKEL CARBONYL
NITROFERRICYANIDES
NONANE
OCTANE
PARAQUAT
PENTACHLOROETHANE
PENTANE
PENTANOL
PETROLEUM ETHERS
POTASSIUM CYANIDE
PROPYL ACETATE
PROPYL ALCOHOLS
PROPYLENE GLYCOL
PROPYLENE OXIDE
QUATERNARY AMMONIUM COMPOUNDS
SODIUM CYANIDE
SODIUM THIOCYANATE

STYRENE
TETRACHLORODIFLUORO-ETHANES
TETRACHLOROETHANES
TETRACHLOROETHYLENE
THIOSULFATES
TOLUENE
TRICHLOROETHANES
TRICHLOROETHYLENE
TRICHLOROTRIFLUORO-ETHANES
TRIETHYLENE GLYCOL
VINYL ACETATE
WHITE SPIRIT
XYLENES

— Never introduce oil or ointment into the eyes without medical advice.

— Notify a physician and inform him of the
- name of the chemical and
- nature of the accident.

---

1. Remove the victim from the source of contamination.
2. Wash affected eye or eyes under slowly running water for 15 minutes or longer, making sure that the victim's eyelids are held wide apart and he moves his eyes slowly in every direction.
3. If pain persists, the medical service will refer the victim to an ophthalmologist and inform him of the nature of the accident and the name of the chemical.
4. If the victim cannot tolerate direct light, protect his eyes with a bandage or handkerchief.

ALKALI DICHROMATES (Ca, K, Na)
ALKALI *META*-BORATES (K, Na)
ALKANES (liquids and solids)
(Alkylmercury compounds)
(Alkyltin compounds)
ALUMINUM CHLORIDE
(Aluminum trichloride)
AMMONIUM CHLORATE
AMMONIUM PERCHLORATE
ARSENIC (soluble salts)
BARIUM (soluble salts)
BARIUM ACETATE
BARIUM CARBONATE
BARIUM CHLORIDE
BARIUM FLUORIDE
BARIUM HYDROXIDE
BARIUM NITRATE
BARIUM OXIDE
BARIUM SULFIDE
BORIC ACID
CALCIUM CHLORIDE
CALCIUM DICHROMATE
CALCIUM HYPOCHLORITE
CHLORINATED LIME
CHLORONAPHTHALENES
CHROMIC ACID
CHROMIUM CHLORIDE
COPPER CHLORIDE
COPPER SULFATE
DIBUTYLLEAD
DIBUTYLTIN
DIETHYLLEAD
DIETHYLMERCURY
DIETHYLTIN
DIHEXYLTIN
DIIODODIETHYLTIN
DIMETHYLMERCURY
DIMETHYLTIN
DIOCTYLTIN
DIPHENYL
DIPHENYLAMINE
DISODIUM PHOSPHATE
ETHYLMERCURY
ETHYLMERCURIC CHLORIDE
ETHYLMERCURIC HYDROXIDE
IRON CHLORIDE
LEAD (metal fumes)
LEAD ACETATE
LEAD ANTIMONATE
LEAD ARSENATE
LEAD CARBONATE
LEAD CHLORIDE
LEAD CHROMATE (red)
LEAD CHROMATE (yellow)
LEAD DIOXIDE
LEAD NITRATE
LEAD OLEATE
LEAD OXIDE (PbO)
LEAD OXIDE (red)
LEAD OXYCHLORIDE
LEAD PHENATE
LEAD PHTHALATE
LEAD STEARATE
LEAD SUBACETATE
LEAD SULFIDE
MAGNESIUM CHLORIDE
MAGNESIUM SULFATE
MERCURIC CHLORIDE
MERCURIC IODIDE
MERCUROUS CHLORIDE
MERCUROUS IODIDE
MERCURY (metal)
MERCURY (organic compounds)
MERCURY (soluble salts)
MERCURY ACETATE
MERCURY FULMINATE
MERCURY NITRATE (acid)
MERCURY OXYCYANIDE
METHYLMERCURY
METHYLMERCURY BORATE
METHYLMERCURY HYDROXIDE
METHYMERCURY IODIDE
METHYLMERCURY NITRATE
METHYLMERCURY PHOSPHATE
NAPHTHALENE
NAPHTHYLAMINES

PARAFFINS (solid compounds)
PERBORATES (K, Na)
PHENYLMERCURIC ACETATE
PEHNYLMERCURY
PHENYLMERCURY OLEATE
PHENYLNAPHTHYLAMINES
PHTHALIC ANHYDRIDE
POTASSIUM BORATE
POTASSIUM CHLORATE
POTASSIUM CHLORIDE
POTASSIUM CHROMATE
POTASSIUM DICHROMATE
POTASSIUM PERCHLORATE
SODIUM BICARBONATE
SODIUM BORATE
SODIUM CHLORATE
SODIUM CHLORIDE
SODIUM CHROMATE
SODIUM DICHROMATE
SODIUM HYPOCHLORITE
SODIUM PERCHLORATE
SODIUM SULFATE
SODIUM THIOSULFATE
TETRABUTYLTIN
TETRAETHYLLEAD
TETRAETHYLTIN
TETRAISOALKYLTINS
TETRAMETHYLLEAD
TETRAPENTYLTIN
TETRAPROPYLTIN
TIN (organic compounds)
TITANIUM CHLORIDES (Tri-, Tetra-)
TRIBUTYLLEAD*
TRIBUTYLTIN*
TRIETHYLLEAD*
TRIETHYLTIN*
TRIMETHYLLEAD*
TRIMETHYLTIN*
TRIPHENYLTIN*
TRIPROPYLTIN*
ZINC CHLORIDE

*probably dimers

— Prevent the victim from rubbing his eyes.

— Never introduce oil or ointment into the eyes without medical advice.

— Notify a physician and inform him of the
  - name of the chemical and
  - nature of the accident.

---

1. Wash the affected eye or eyes under slowly running water for 15 minutes or longer, making sure that the victim's eyelids are held wide apart and he moves his eyes slowly in every direction.
2. Make sure that no solid particles of the chemical remain in the creases of the eye; if they do, continue to wash the eye.
3. If the pain persists, the medical service will refer the victim to an ophthalmologist and inform him of the nature of the chemical.

IN CASE OF EYE CONTACT WITH

ALUMINUM (dust)
(Aluminum hydrate)
ALUMINUM HYDROXIDE
ALUMINUM OXIDE
ASBESTOS
CALCIUM CARBONATE
CARBON
CARBON BLACK
KAOLIN
POLY(VINYL CHLORIDE)
SILICA
TALC
TITANIUM (dust)
TITANIUM OXIDE
TUNGSTEN CARBIDE

— Prevent the victim from rubbing his eyes.

Accompany the victim to the dispensary where the eyes will be rinsed.

NOTE: In case irritating particles are found in the eye, the physician will refer the victim to an ophthalmologist and inform him of the nature of the accident and the chemical.

IN CASE OF EYE CONTACT WITH

(Alkylaluminum compounds)
ALUMINUM ALKYLS
DIETHYLALUMINUM CHLORIDE
DIETHYLALUMINUM HYDRIDE
TRIETHYLALUMINUM
TRIISOBUTYLALUMINUM
TRIMETHYLALUMINUM

— Notify a physician immediately and inform him of the
- name of the chemical and
- nature of the accident.

1. Make sure the victim does not run away.
2. Wash the victim's head **immediately** with plenty of water, if possible with a hand-held hose. (The flames will increase in intensity when water is first applied but will then die out.)
3. Lay the victim flat on his back on a stretcher and cover his eyes with a clean bandage.
4. Take him immediately to the hospital.

IN CASE OF EYE CONTACT WITH

CHLORTHION
DDVP
DEMETON
DIAZINON
DIPTEREX
EPN
ISOPESTOX
MALATHION
METHYL PARATHION
OMPA
ORGANOPHOSPHORUS COMPOUNDS
PARAOXON
PARATHION
PHOSDRIN
PHOSPHORIC ESTERS
RONNEL
SULFOTEPP
TEPP
TRITHION

— It is vital to apply first aid without delay.

— In all instances, even MILD CASES, notify a physician immediately of the
  - name of the chemical and
  - nature of the accident.

— Never introduce oil or ointment into the eyes.

---

1. Remove the victim from the source of contamination and take him immediately to the nearest eye wash or shower.
2. Quickly wipe any excess chemical from his face.
3. Immediately wash the affected eye or eyes under slowly running water for 15 minutes or longer, making sure that the victim's eyelids are held wide apart and he moves his eyes slowly in every direction.

If the victim is conscious but has difficulty in breathing,

1. Lay him on his back with his head lowered and his legs raised.
2. Loosen his collar and belt.
3. Cover him with a blanket.
4. Make him inhale oxygen until the doctor arrives.

In the case of the above symptoms, the physician **should be called immediately to treat the victim**.

APPENDIX A
GENERAL INSTRUCTIONS IN CASE OF POISONING BY UNKNOWN CHEMICAL PRODUCTS

It is relatively rare in most situations where chemicals are being handled not to know the exact nature of the substance that has caused poisoning or an accident.

These instructions are applicable in all those cases where the identity of the substance concerned is unknown.

1. Try to determine
   a. the exact nature of the toxic substance that caused the poisoning or accident.
   b. the way in which the harmful substance has contaminated the victim by examining the site of the accident, followed by a quick examination of the lips, mucous membranes of the mouth, tongue, the state of integuments, and the circumstances. Palpation of a distended abdomen that causes pain is proof of ingestion of a corrosive or caustic substance.
2. Notify a physician immediately and inform him of the state of the victim and of the probable nature of the substance, if this is known.

A. POISONING BY INHALATION

In the case of high contamination, the first aider should wear a self-contained mask before entering the suspect area.

1. Assess the condition of the poisoned victim and take note of the state of the premises and any abnormal features (smell, fumes, dust) to try to identify the toxic vapors; then refer to the name of the substance in the INDEX and check the symptoms on the **white** pages.
   In every case, remove the victim as soon as possible from the contaminated area and lay him down in a cool, quiet, well-ventilated area.
2. **If the victim has stopped breathing,** begin artificial respiration immediately in the fresh air (HOLGER-NIELSEN method or mouth-to-mouth resuscitation with an AMBU-type bellow*). **Never use direct mouth-to-mouth resuscitation if the nature of the toxic substance is unknown.**
3. **Never give an unconscious victim anything to drink** (danger of suffocation or pneumonia).

B. POISONING BY INGESTION

The state of the lips and mouth may indicate a case of ingestion even if the victim has lost consciousness.

1. **If the victim has stopped breathing,** lay him on his stomach and use normal artificial respiration by the HOLGER-NIELSEN method or with an AMBU-type bellow,* while awaiting the arrival of a resuscitator of the PULMOTOR, PNEOPHORE, PORTON, or AIROX type.*
2. **If the victim is unconscious but breathing, never try to make him drink or vomit.**
   Lay him with his head lowered in a cool room while awaiting the physician's arrival.
   Do not forget to remove dentures or partial plates!
3. **If the victim is conscious,** try to get rid of the toxic substance by making him vomit. Ask him to stick two fingers down his throat or tickle his uvula carefully with the handle of a spoon. Lower his head so that he cannot inhale the vomited substance. (Exceptions to this

*See Vital Equipment, page 4.

rule are strong acids, caustic substances, and HYDROGEN PEROXIDE where it is preferable not to induce vomiting to prevent additional burning of the esophagus and the larynx.) Afterwards, give the victim plenty of water to drink.

4. Always keep the vomit for possible analysis.
5. Notify the physician and inform him of the circumstances of the poisoning and the state of the victim. In every case, ask for an adequate oxygen apparatus.*
6. Quickly carry out investigations to determine the exact nature of the substance (by analyzing the urine, vomit, or remaining substance).
7. Prevent a state of shock
   - weak and rapid pulse
   - cold sweat—pale complexion
   - tendency to fainting
   - cold hands and feet

   by covering the victim with a blanket or warm clothes.
8. **If the victim shows signs of shock,** lay him on his back, with his head lowered and his legs raised until the color returns to his face and his pulse becomes stronger.

C. POISONING BY SKIN CONTACT

1. In all cases where chemicals splash onto the skin, remove contaminated clothing as quickly as possible and wash the affected areas very gently under running water (shower), keeping the eyes protected and treating the skin, which may be inflamed, carefully. The first aiders must take precautions not to introduce corrosive substance into their eyes (protective goggles must be worn).
2. Make sure that the victim does not catch cold after the shower; dress him in dry clothes or wrap him in a clean blanket while awaiting the physician's arrival.

*See Vital Equipment, page 4.

D. POISONING BY SPLASHING IN THE EYES

Immediate action is vital.

1. Take the victim immediately to an eye wash or to a shower, wash his eyes and make sure that the eyelids are held wide apart; continue washing for at least 15 minutes, while asking him to move his eyes in every direction.
2. **Never introduce oil or greasy ointment into the eyes without medical advice.**
3. Always refer the victim to an opthalmologist.

APPENDIX B
U.S. GOVERNMENT PUBLICATIONS

The U.S. government has published various documents relative to occupational safety and health of workers exposed to a number of compounds in commerce. These documents are valuable for the scope of their treatment of the toxicology, origins, and other matters relating to the compounds named. Copies of these documents may be obtained from the Superintendent of Documents, U.S. Government Printing Office, Washington, D.C. 20402. Since new documents are being issued and old ones updated and reissued, it is important and worthwhile to write NIOSH for all newly issued documents.

Compounds listed in this book have been described in the following lists of publications by National Institute for Occupational Safety (NIOSH), Publications Dissemination, Division of Technical Services, 4676 Columbia Parkway, Cincinnati, Ohio 45226.

CURRENT INTELLIGENCE BULLETINS

Chloroethanes, No. 27
Vinyl Bromide, Vinyl Chloride, and Vinylidene Chloride, No. 28

CRITERIA FOR RECOMMENDED STANDARDS
FOR OCCUPATIONAL EXPOSURE.

Acetylene
Alkanes (C_5–C_8)
Allyl Chloride
Ammonia
Arsenic
Asbestos

Benzene
Boron Trifluoride
Cadmium
Carbon Black
Carbon Dioxide
Carbon Disulfide
Carbon Monoxide
Carbon Tetrachloride
Chlorine
Chloroethanes
Chloroform
Chromic Acid
Chromium (VI)
Crystalline Silica
Dinitro-*o*-cresol
Epichlorohydrin
Ethylene Dichloride
Formaldehyde
Glycidyl Ethers
Hydrogen Cyanide and Cyanide Salts
Hydrogen Fluoride
Hydrogen Sulfide
Inorganic Arsenic
Inorganic Fluoride
Inorganic Lead
Inorganic Mercury
Inorganic Nickel
Isopropyl Alcohol
Malathion
Methyl Alcohol
Methylene Chloride
Methyl Parathion
Nitric Acid
Nitrogen
Nitroglycerin and Ethylene Glycol Dinitrate
Organo-tin
Parathion
Phenol
Sodium Hydroxide
Sulfur Dioxide
Sulfuric Acid
1,1,2,2-Tetrachloroethane
Toluene
Trichloroethylene and Methyl Chloroform
Vinyl Chloride
Xylene
Zinc Oxide

APPENDIX C
GLOSSARY OF COMMERCIAL NAMES

Commercial Name	*Chemical Name*
CLORTHION	*0,0*-Dimethyl *0*-(3-chloro-4-nitrophenyl) thionophosphate
DDVP	*0,0*-Dimethyl *0*-(2,2-dichlorovinyl) phosphate
DEMETON	*0,0*-Diethyl *0*-(2-ethylthioethyl) thionophosphate mixed with *0,0*-diethyl *S*-[2-(ethylthio)ethyl] phosphorothioate
DIAZINON	*0,0*-Diethyl *0*-[6-methyl-2-(1-methylethyl)-4-pyrimidinyl] phosphorothioate
DIPTEREX	*0,0*-Dimethyl 2,2,2-trichloro-1-hydroxyethylphosphonate
DIQUAT	6,7-Dihydrodipyrido[1,2-a:2′,1′-c] pyrazinediium dibromide
DNBP	2-*sec*-Butyl-4,6-dinitrophenol
DNOC	4,6-Dinitro-*o*-cresol
EPN	*0*-Ethyl *0*-*p*-nitrophenyl phenylphosphonothioate
GRAMOXON	1,1′-Dimethyl-4,4′-bipyridinium dichloride
ISOPESTOX	*N,N′*-Diisopropylphosphorodiamidic fluoride
MALATHION	*S*-(1,2-Dicarboxyethyl) *0,0*-dimethyl phosphorothioate

METHYL PARATHION	*0,0*-Dimethyl *0-p*-nitrophenyl phosphorothioate
OMPA	Octamethylpyrophosphoramide
PARAOXON	*0,0*-Diethyl *0-p*-nitrophenyl phosphate
PARAQUAT	1,1′-Dimethyl-4,4′-bipyridinium dichloride
PARATHION	*0,0*-Diethyl *0-p*-nitrophenyl phosphorothioate
PHOSDRIN	3-[(Dimethoxyphosphinyl)oxy]-2-butenoic acid methyl ester
RONNEL	*0,0*-Dimethyl *0*-(2,4,5-trichlorophenyl) phosphorothioate
SULFOTEPP	Tetraethyl thiopyrophosphate
TEPP	Tetraethyl pyrophosphate
TRITHION	*0,0*-Diethyl *S*-[[(4-chlorophenyl)thio]methyl] phosphorodithioate